EART

"The Hidden Power of Grounding"

HARKEEM SHAW

COPYRIGHT© 2023

All rights reserved.

No part of this book may be reproduced in any form or by any electronic or mechanical means, including information storage and retrieval systems, without written permission from the author, except for the use of brief quotations in a book review.

First edition

Although the author and publisher have made every effort to ensure that the information in this book was correct at press time, the author and publisher do not assume and hereby disclaim any liability to any party for any lost, damage, or disruption caused by error or omission, whether such error or omissions result from negligence, accident, or any other cause. Likewise, the author and publisher assume no responsibilities for any false information. No liability is assumed for damages that may result from the reading or use of information contained within.

CONTENTS

1. Grounding and the Immune System 6
2. Grounding and Emotional Well-being 9
3. Grounding and Sleep 12
4. Grounding and Stress Reduction 15
5. Grounding and Athletic Performance 18
6. Grounding and Environment al Sustainability 21
7. Grounding and Children's Health 27
8. Grounding and Workplace Wellness 30
9. Grounding and Mindfulness 33
10. Grounding and Energy Medicine 36
11. Grounding and Environmental Conservation 39
12. Grounding and Spiritual Growth 43
13. Grounding and Digestive Health 47
14. Grounding and Skin Health 50
15. Grounding and Hormonal Balance 53
16. Grounding and Brain Health 56
17. Grounding and Heart Health 59
18. Grounding and Environmental Justice 62
19. Grounding and the Gut-Brain Axis 65
20. Grounding and Social Connection 68
21. Grounding and the Power of Visualization 72
22. Grounding and the Power of Affirmations 75
23. Grounding and the Power of Crystals 78
24. Grounding and the Power of Breathwork 81

25. Grounding and the Power of Yoga 84
26. Grounding and the Power of Meditation.......................... 88
27. Grounding and the Power of Massage Therapy 92
28. Grounding and the Power of Sound Healing...................... 96
29. Grounding and the Power of Herbal Medicine 100
30. Grounding and the Power of Reiki 103
31. Grounding and the Power of Ayurveda........................... 107
32. Grounding and the Power of Energy Psychology............. 111
33. Grounding and the Power of Mind-Body-Spirit Connection.. 115
34. Grounding and the Power of Community 119
35. Grounding and the Power of Nature Immersion............... 122
36. Grounding and the Power of Forest Bathing..................... 126
37. Grounding and the Power of Water................................. 130
38. Grounding and the Power of Sunlight............................. 134
39. Grounding and the Power of Breath of Fresh Air............. 137
40. Grounding and the Power of Sacred Spaces..................... 140
41. Grounding and the Power of Journaling 143
42. Grounding and the Power of Art Therapy....................... 146
43. Grounding and the Power of Dance 150
44. Grounding and Addiction Recovery 153
45. Grounding and Trauma Healing 156
46. Grounding and the Power of Mind-Body Connection...... 159
47. Grounding and the Power of Intention............................ 162
48. Grounding and the Power of Affection 165
49. Grounding and the Power of Self-Care........................... 169

50. Grounding and the Power of Self-Compassion 173
51. Grounding and the Power of Forgiveness 177
52. Grounding and the Power of Gratitude 180
53. Grounding and the Power of Connection 183
54. Grounding and the Power of Empathy................................ 187
55. Grounding and the Power of Boundaries 191
56. Grounding and the Power of Creativity.............................. 195
57. Grounding and the Power of Movement 199
58. Grounding and the Power of Nutrition................................ 202
59. Grounding and the Power of Mindful Eating 206
60. Grounding and the Power of Mindful Communication ... 209
61. Grounding and the Power of Mindful Parenting................ 212
62. Grounding and the Power of Mindful Leadership 216
63. Grounding and the Power of Mindful Technology Use ... 220
64. Grounding and the Power of Mindful Travel 223
65. Grounding and the Power of Mindful Aging..................... 227
66. Grounding and Addiction Recover....................................... 230
67. Grounding and Trauma Healing.. 233
68. Grounding and the Power of Mind-Body Connection 236
69. Grounding and the Power of Intention 239
70. Grounding and the Power of Affection............................... 242
71. Grounding and the Power of Self-Care............................... 245
72. Grounding and the Power of Self-Compassion 248
73. Grounding and the Power of Forgiveness 251
74. Grounding and the Power of Gratitude 254
75. Grounding and the Power of Connection 257

76. Grounding and the Power of Empathy 260
77. Grounding and the Power of Boundaries 263
78. Grounding and the Power of Creativity.............................. 266
79. Grounding and the Power of Movement 269
80. Grounding and the Power of Nutrition 272
81. Grounding and the Power of Mindful Eating.................... 275
82. Grounding and the Power of Mindful Communication ... 278
83. Grounding and the Power of Mindful Parenting 281
84. Grounding and the Power of Mindful Leadership............ 285
85. Grounding and the Power of Mindful Technology Use ... 289
Here Is A List Of Illnesses That Grounding May Potentially Be Beneficial 292
Debunking Myths: Clearing Misconceptions
about Grounding 367
Testimonial.. 370
Frequently ask Questions 381
Dictionary 384
References... 410
About The Author.. 410

DEDICATION

First, I would like to give thanks to the almighty God for guiding me with wisdom and directing me to create this insightful book. To my mom, Janice Shaw, who was always there to guide me in spirit and help me through the whole journey. I am doing this for her and my lovely daughter, Marlisa Shaw. I value my daughter as my strength. Indeed, you both have been my biggest inspiration. I would like to give a big thanks to my family and friends, without you, this book would not have been its best.

INTRODUCTION TO GROUNDING

Grounding is a therapeutic technique that involves connecting the body to the natural electrical properties of the Earth. The idea is that by putting our bodies into contact with the Earth's surface through grounding, we can get a variety of benefits that can improve our overall health and well-being. In this section, we will explore the concept of Grounding and its benefits in detail.

What is Grounding?

Grounding is a technique that involves connecting the body to the Earth's surface. This can be done by walking barefoot on the ground, lying on the grass, or using Grounding products that are designed to mimic the Earth's electrical properties. The Earth's surface has a natural electrical charge, and when we come into contact with it, we can absorb this charge into our bodies.

The Benefits of Grounding

Grounding has been shown to have a variety of benefits for our health and well-being. Some of the benefits of Grounding include:

Reduced inflammation: Grounding has been shown to reduce inflammation in the body, which can help alleviate symptoms of chronic pain and other inflammatory conditions.

Inflammation: it's a natural and vital part of our body's defense mechanism, playing a critical role in healing and protecting us from injuries and infections. However, when inflammation becomes chronic or out of balance, it can lead to numerous health problems and negatively impact our quality of life. Recent research suggests that grounding, or earthing, can reduce inflammation and alleviate symptoms of various inflammatory conditions. Grounding refers to the simple yet profound practice of reconnecting with the Earth's surface. The Earth's surface maintains a negative charge, abundant with free electrons. When our bodies, barefoot or otherwise directly connected to the Earth, these electrons are absorbed, offering a range of health benefits. One of the most significant benefits is reduced inflammation.

The Science of Grounding and Inflammation

To understand how grounding reduces inflammation, we first need to look at what happens during inflammation at the cellular level. When tissues are damaged by injuries, toxins, or infections, the body responds by releasing substances that trigger inflammation to protect and heal the affected area. These substances include free radicals, unstable molecules with an unpaired electron, causing them to seek out other electrons to become stable, damaging cells in the process. This 'oxidative stress' can result in further inflammation, perpetuating a damaging cycle.

Grounding works by providing a rich source of electrons from the Earth, which can neutralize these harmful free radicals, stabilizing them and preventing them from causing further cellular damage. In essence, the Earth's electrons act as natural antioxidants. This process is believed to break the cycle of oxidative stress and inflammation, allowing the body to heal more effectively.

In a groundbreaking study by Gaétan Chevalier and his colleagues, published in the Journal of Inflammation Research, grounding was found to reduce inflammation and promote wound healing. In the study, participants who were grounded had less redness, swelling, and heat - classic signs of inflammation - around a wound than those who were not. This research provided visual evidence that grounding could indeed reduce inflammation.

Practical Implications: Grounding and Chronic Inflammatory Conditions

Chronic inflammation is believed to play a central role in many health conditions, including heart disease, diabetes, arthritis, and certain cancers. It's also linked to autoimmune disorders, allergies, and even neurological disorders like depression and Alzheimer's disease. By reducing inflammation, grounding holds potential in managing these conditions and improving overall health.

For example, arthritis, characterized by chronic inflammation in the joints leading to pain and stiffness, could potentially be managed through grounding practices. Similarly, grounding may alleviate inflammation-related pain in conditions like **fibromyalgia** or **chronic back pain**.

Grounding has also been shown to help reduce muscle soreness and accelerate recovery in athletes, largely due to its anti-inflammatory effects. In a study by Brown et al., grounding was found to reduce blood markers of muscle damage and inflammation in participants who had completed a strenuous exercise.

Furthermore, grounding's impact on reducing inflammation could potentially extend to mental health. Inflammation has been linked to depression, anxiety, and stress. By reducing inflammation, grounding could potentially help improve mood and reduce anxiety.

Finally, it's important to consider that grounding is a natural, cost-free, and accessible practice that can be easily incorporated into daily life. Whether by walking barefoot in a park, sitting on a grounded mat, or using a grounding sheet, practice offers a promising approach to health and wellness.

It's important to note that while grounding holds immense potential, it should not replace medical treatments or interventions for inflammatory conditions. Individuals with chronic illnesses should consult their healthcare providers before making any significant changes to their treatment plans.

In conclusion, grounding provides a promising avenue for reducing inflammation and associated health conditions. As research continues to explore this exciting field, grounding's potential in improving health and well-being becomes increasingly apparent. With the simplicity and accessibility of grounding, it's a practice we could all consider incorporating into our daily lives for its profound benefits.

1. GROUNDING AND THE IMMUNE SYSTEM

Investigating the impact of Grounding on immune function and overall health.

The immune system, a complex network of cells, organs, and biological responses, serves as our body's primary defense mechanism against harmful pathogens and diseases. In an era of increasing health concerns, particularly those that stem from immune dysfunction, strategies that can naturally and effectively bolster our immune health are of vital interest. One such strategy, known as grounding or earthing, is gaining recognition for its potential to enhance immune function and promote overall health.

Understanding the Immune System

Before exploring the relationship between grounding and immune health, it is essential to understand the basic functions of the immune system. The immune system serves two primary roles: recognizing and neutralizing harmful pathogens and repairing tissue damage caused by injury or disease. Both of these roles involve complex cellular and molecular processes that can lead to inflammation and oxidative stress, two chronic states that can compromise immune health and lead to a variety of health problems.

Grounding and its Impact on Inflammation

Grounding's potential to enhance immune health primarily lies in its ability to counteract inflammation. By making direct, skin-to-surface contact with the Earth, our bodies can absorb the Earth's free electrons. These free electrons have antioxidant properties, neutralizing the free radicals that contribute to the inflammatory process. In this way, grounding can regulate the immune response, preventing overactivity that could otherwise lead to chronic inflammation and various inflammatory conditions.

Regulating Oxidative Stress Through Grounding

Oxidative stress, characterized by an overabundance of free radicals, is another mechanism through which the immune system can be compromised. By providing an external source of free electrons, grounding can help neutralize excess free radicals, reducing oxidative stress and protecting cells from oxidative damage. This not only aids the immune system in repairing damaged tissues but also helps maintain the integrity and function of immune cells, enabling them to effectively respond to harmful pathogens.

Promoting Healing and Recovery

The immune-enhancing effects of grounding also extend to the body's healing and recovery processes. By reducing inflammation and oxidative stress, grounding can create an environment conducive to healing, accelerating tissue repair and wound healing. This can be particularly beneficial following injury, surgery, or in conditions that impair the body's natural healing capabilities.

Grounding and Immune-Related Conditions

Grounding's immune-boosting properties can have significant implications for various health conditions associated with immune dysfunction. These include autoimmune conditions, in which the immune system mistakenly attacks the body's cells, and immunodeficiency disorders, where the immune system's ability to fight off infections is compromised. By regulating immune responses, grounding can potentially alleviate symptoms, improve quality of life, and reduce the risk of complications associated with these conditions.

Incorporating Grounding into Everyday Life

There are numerous ways to incorporate grounding into your daily routine, whether it be walking barefoot outside, swimming in natural water bodies, or using grounding equipment such as grounding mats, sheets, or bands. Regular grounding practices, when combined with a balanced diet, regular exercise, and sufficient sleep, can significantly contribute to optimal immune function and overall health.

Conclusion

Grounding, an age-old practice grounded in scientific principles, offers a promising, accessible, and natural strategy for enhancing immune health. As research into the health benefits of grounding continues to evolve, it is becoming increasingly clear that our connection to the Earth can serve as a powerful tool in maintaining and improving our health, reinforcing the notion that nature, in its simplicity and wisdom, holds many of the answers to our health and wellbeing.

2. GROUNDING AND EMOTIONAL WELL-BEING

Discussing how Grounding practices can support emotional balance and mental well-being.

In a world increasingly characterized by stress, anxiety, and emotional imbalance, strategies that promote mental well-being are vital. One practice gaining attention in the realm of emotional health is grounding, or earthing, which connects us physically to the Earth. Emerging research suggests that grounding can significantly impact emotional well-being, offering a natural and accessible tool for enhancing emotional health and overall quality of life.

Understanding Emotional Well-being

Emotional well-being refers to the ability to successfully manage emotions, maintain positive relationships, and effectively cope with life's challenges. It is an essential component of our overall health, influencing our thoughts, behaviors, physical health, and life quality. Emotional well-being is not merely the absence of mental health disorders but a state of positive emotional health and resilience.

Grounding and Stress Reduction

One of the key ways Grounding can support emotional well-being is by reducing stress. Stress is a common feature of modern life and can have detrimental effects on our physical and emotional health if not properly managed. Grounding can influence the autonomic nervous system, shifting it towards a state of relaxation and reducing the production of cortisol, a hormone released in response to stress. This helps to mitigate the harmful effects of chronic stress and promote a sense of calm and tranquility.

Enhancing Mood and Alleviating Anxiety

Grounding's calming effects can also lead to enhanced mood and reduced anxiety. By promoting physiological relaxation, grounding can help ease feelings of tension, worry, and restlessness often associated with anxiety. Furthermore, the physical act of connecting with nature through grounding can also improve mood, promoting feelings of joy and contentment.

Promoting Sleep and Circadian Rhythm Regulation

Good quality sleep is integral to emotional well-being, with sleep deprivation often leading to mood disorders, anxiety, and reduced stress resilience. Grounding can help regulate our natural sleep-wake cycle, or circadian rhythm, promoting deeper and more restful sleep. This can lead to enhanced emotional stability, improved mood, and better cognitive function, all of which contribute to emotional well-being.

Grounding as a Mindfulness Practice

Grounding can also serve as a form of mindfulness practice, which is known to support emotional well-being. By focusing our attention on the physical sensation of connecting with the Earth, we can anchor ourselves in the present moment, reducing rumination on past events or worries about the future. This mindful aspect of grounding can enhance emotional awareness, improve stress management, and promote a state of mental calm and clarity.

Conclusion

The practice of grounding offers a simple yet potent tool for supporting emotional well-being. Its ability to reduce stress, enhance mood, promote restful sleep, and foster mindfulness can significantly contribute to emotional balance and resilience. As we continue to navigate an ever-complex world, grounding provides an accessible path to emotional well-being, reconnecting us with nature's healing power and reminding us of our inherent capacity for emotional health and harmony.

3. GROUNDING AND SLEEP

Exploring the connection between Grounding and improved sleep quality and regulation

The significance of sleep cannot be overstated. It is a crucial component of our overall health, playing a pivotal role in various biological processes, including cellular repair, cognitive function, and emotional well-being. In our hectic, always-connected modern lives, quality sleep is often compromised, leading to a host of physical and mental health issues. As we seek solutions to improve sleep quality, one natural approach, known as grounding or earthing, has emerged with promising potential.

Understanding Sleep and Its Importance

Sleep isn't simply a time of rest or inactivity. It's an active period during which a variety of essential processing, restoration, and strengthening processes occur. Our bodies require long periods of sleep to restore and rejuvenate, to grow muscle, repair tissue, and synthesize hormones.

In addition, sleep is essential for our cognitive functions such as memory, learning, creativity, and problem-solving. It also plays a vital role in our emotional health and wellbeing, influencing our mood, resilience to stress, and even our relationships with others.

The Concept of Grounding

Grounding, also known as earthing, is a therapeutic technique that focuses on realigning our bodies' electrical energy by reconnecting us to the Earth's surface. It is based on the principle that our bodies are made up of electrical ions and that, without a stable influx of electrons from the Earth's surface, we can become susceptible to inflammation, circadian rhythm disorders, hormonal imbalances, and other health complications.

The Impact of Grounding on Sleep

Grounding's potential for improving sleep lies in its influence over the nervous system and hormone production, primarily cortisol, the so-called 'stress hormone.' Here's how:

Regulation of Cortisol Production: One of the most significant findings around grounding is its effect on cortisol production. Cortisol follows a natural rhythm throughout the day, with levels typically peaking in the morning to wake us up and gradually declining throughout the day to lowest at night, allowing us to sleep. This is known as the cortisol awakening response (CAR). However, stress, among other factors, can disrupt this rhythm. Irregular cortisol levels, particularly when high at night, are linked to sleep disturbances. Grounding has been shown to help normalize cortisol production, thus aiding the regulation of sleep.

Autonomic Nervous System Balance

The Autonomic Nervous System (ANS) controls many of our body's functions, including heart rate, digestion, and—pertinently—our sleep-wake cycle. The ANS is composed of two branches: the sympathetic nervous system (SNS), which initiates the 'fight or flight' response, and the parasympathetic nervous system (PNS), which encourages the 'rest and digest' state. Grounding is suggested to promote a shift towards PNS dominance, thus encouraging relaxation and sleep.

Reduction in Pain and Inflammation

Pain and inflammation can significantly impair sleep quality. The anti-inflammatory effects of grounding, which are thought to result from the influx of negatively charged electrons neutralizing positively charged free radicals, can help reduce pain and promote more restful sleep.

Grounding Practices for Improved Sleep

Integrating grounding into our routines can be as simple as spending time barefoot outside on natural surfaces like grass, sand, or soil. However, for many, such regular contact with nature might be impractical. Fortunately, grounding can also be achieved through the use of grounding mats or sheets, which are connected to the Earth via a wire plugged into a grounded wall outlet or a rod placed in the ground outside.

These grounding tools can be used while sleeping, thus providing the benefits of grounding throughout the night and potentially improving sleep quality and duration. It's worth noting, however, that grounding mats and sheets should be used in conjunction with a holistic sleep hygiene regimen to yield the most significant benefits.

Conclusion

As research into grounding continues to emerge, its potential for improving sleep presents a compelling case for the practice. With its influences on cortisol production, the autonomic nervous system, and inflammation, grounding offers a natural and accessible tool for supporting sleep health. While grounding is not a substitute for good sleep hygiene and medical advice, it can form part of a holistic approach to improving sleep quality and overall health.

4. GROUNDING AND STRESS REDUCTION

Examining how Grounding practices can help reduce stress and promote relaxation.

In an era marked by increasing digitalization, constant connectivity, and unrelenting demands on our time, stress has become an omnipresent challenge. Chronic stress not only detrimentally impacts our mental well-being but also our physical health, contributing to various disorders like hypertension, diabetes, and cardiovascular diseases. As society grapples with this stress epidemic, grounding – a practice that draws us back to our connection with nature – is gaining traction for its potential stress-reducing benefits.

Understanding Stress and its Impact

Stress is a biological response to demanding circumstances, activating the body's 'fight or flight' system to cope with perceived threats. While this reaction is beneficial in acute, short-term scenarios, chronic stress is harmful. Prolonged activation of the stress response system can disrupt almost all body processes, increasing the risk of numerous health problems.

Grounding and Stress Reduction

Several mechanisms underline the stress-reducing potential of grounding, including:

Regulation of the Autonomic Nervous System (ANS): The ANS controls many body processes, including the body's stress response. Grounding has been shown to promote the 'rest and digest' activities associated with the parasympathetic nervous system, the calming branch of the ANS, reducing the hyperactivity of the sympathetic nervous system, the 'fight or flight' branch.

Balancing Cortisol Levels: Cortisol, the 'stress hormone', follows a natural daily rhythm, peaking in the morning and declining throughout the day. Chronic stress disrupts this rhythm, leading to elevated nighttime cortisol and associated sleep disturbances. Research suggests that grounding can help normalize cortisol levels, thereby reducing stress and improving sleep.

Reduction in Inflammation and Pain: Chronic inflammation, often caused by ongoing stress, is associated with numerous health conditions. Grounding is thought to neutralize free radicals, unstable molecules causing inflammation and cell damage, through an influx of negatively charged electrons. By reducing inflammation and associated pain, grounding can contribute to stress relief.

Improved Sleep and Mood: Sleep disturbances and mood disorders are often both causes and effects of chronic stress. By regulating cortisol production and promoting a more balanced sleep-wake cycle, grounding can help improve mood and reduce symptoms of anxiety and depression, contributing to overall stress reduction.

Incorporating Grounding into Daily Life

Incorporating grounding into our routines can be as simple as spending time barefoot outside on natural surfaces like grass or sand. However, for those living in urban environments or cold climates, direct contact with the Earth may be impractical.

Fortunately, grounding can also be achieved using grounding mats, sheets, or bands, which connect to the Earth's natural charge via a grounded wall outlet, or a rod placed in the ground outside.

It's essential to note that grounding should be viewed as a supplementary tool for stress reduction and not a replacement for other proven stress management techniques such as regular exercise, a healthy diet, and adequate sleep.

Conclusion

While scientific research on grounding is still in its early stages, preliminary findings, along with a wealth of anecdotal reports, suggest that grounding may offer a valuable tool for stress reduction. As part of a holistic approach to stress management, grounding may help mitigate the effects of our increasingly hectic, digitally dominated lifestyles, fostering greater relaxation and well-being.

5. GROUNDING AND ATHLETIC PERFORMANCE

Investigating the potential benefits of Grounding for athletes and physical performance.

The sporting world is always on the lookout for novel techniques that can enhance athletic performance, accelerate recovery, and reduce injury risk. Grounding, also known as earthing, is one such method that has garnered attention. This practice, which involves making direct contact with the Earth's surface, is being explored for its potential benefits in boosting athletic performance and recovery.

The Physiology of Exercise and Recovery

To understand the impact of grounding on athletic performance, it is crucial to grasp the physiological processes involved in exercise and recovery. When an athlete engages in strenuous physical activity, it generates a metabolic response that includes the production of free radicals. Although these molecules play essential roles in cell signaling and homeostasis, an excessive amount can cause oxidative stress, leading to inflammation and tissue damage, manifesting as fatigue, reduced performance, and extended recovery times.

Potential Benefits of Grounding for Athletic Performance

Research into the effects of grounding on athletic performance and recovery is still in its infancy, but initial studies and anecdotal reports suggest several potential benefits:

Reduced Muscle Damage and Inflammation

Some studies suggest that grounding may reduce muscle damage and inflammation following strenuous exercise. These effects are thought to be due to the influx of electrons from the Earth, which can neutralize excess free radicals produced during intense physical activity.

Improved Sleep and Recovery

Sleep is an essential component of athletic recovery. It is during sleep that the body repairs muscle tissue and consolidates memory, including motor skills learned during training. Grounding has been shown to improve sleep quality, which could, in turn, enhance recovery and subsequent performance.

Pain Reduction

Several athletes who use grounding techniques have reported reduced pain following injuries or intense training sessions. Again, this is likely due to the reduction in inflammation that grounding can promote.

Enhanced Parasympathetic Activation

Grounding may enhance the activation of the parasympathetic nervous system - the branch of the autonomic nervous system responsible for 'rest and digest' activities. Increased parasympathetic activity is associated with better recovery, as it promotes relaxation, digestion, and tissue repair.

Improved Mood and Reduced Stress

Grounding has been associated with improved mood and reduced stress. Athletic performance can be influenced by both mood and stress levels. A positive mood can boost motivation, while lower stress levels can improve focus and skill execution. Grounding Techniques for Athletes

Incorporating grounding into an athlete's routine can be as simple as spending time barefoot outside on natural surfaces, such as grass, sand, or soil. However, practicality or climate may sometimes make this challenging. Grounding mats, sheets, and bands provide alternatives, allowing athletes to ground themselves indoors.

It's essential to remember that while grounding presents potential benefits, it does not replace a balanced diet, regular training, adequate hydration, and sleep – all critical components of athletic performance and recovery.

The Future of Grounding in Sports

As the scientific community continues to investigate grounding, it is hoped that a clearer picture of its impact on athletic performance and recovery will emerge. Current evidence, although preliminary, is encouraging, suggesting that grounding could offer a valuable addition to athletes' toolkit.

Overall, grounding represents an intersection between ancient wisdom and modern science. The method encourages a return to our natural connection with the Earth, a connection that may offer an array of benefits for athletes and non-athletes alike. As we continue to explore and understand these benefits, grounding may well become a standard part of sports training and recovery protocols in the future.

6. GROUNDING AND ENVIRONMENTAL SUSTAINABILITY

Discussing how Grounding practices can foster a deeper connection with nature and promote environmental awareness.

In our technologically advanced, fast-paced world, humans have, in many ways, become disconnected from the natural environments from which they originated. Practices like grounding (or earthing) provide a bridge back to our inherent connection with the Earth and could play a pivotal role in fostering a deeper appreciation for nature and enhancing environmental sustainability.

Grounding and Connection to Nature

When we engage in grounding, we interact with the Earth in an intimate, physical way that transcends our usual experiences. As our skin contacts the Earth's surface, we can better appreciate our kinship with the natural world, recognizing that we are part of an interconnected web of life.

Such experiences can help dissolve the perceived barriers between 'us' and 'nature,' reminding us that we are not separate entities observing the environment from afar but integral components of the ecosystem. By fostering this deeper connection to nature, grounding can stimulate more conscious thought about our actions and their impact on the environment.

Promoting Environmental Awareness

Grounding has the potential to act as a catalyst for environmental awareness and sustainable behavior. Practice encourages us to slow down, step outside, and immerse ourselves in the natural environment, which can evoke a sense of awe and respect for the world around us.

As we experience the potential health benefits of grounding, we might feel gratitude towards the Earth and its healing properties. This gratitude can engender a sense of responsibility and a desire to preserve the environment, prompting more eco-friendly behaviors.

Grounding as an Act of Environmental Stewardship

Grounding can be viewed as an act of environmental stewardship. As we practice grounding, we benefit directly from the Earth's resources, reminding us of the importance of preserving these resources for future generations. The act of grounding can become symbolic, representing our commitment to sustainable practices and environmental care.

Moreover, as grounding becomes a regular practice, it may naturally lead individuals to spend more time outdoors, potentially participating in outdoor preservation activities such as tree planting, litter clean-ups, and community gardening. These activities can contribute to the overall health of our local ecosystems while enhancing our connection to the Earth.

Grounding in an Era of Environmental Crisis

In an era of environmental crisis, practices that promote a deep connection to the Earth, like grounding, are of immense value. As we face challenges like climate change, deforestation, and pollution, grounding reminds us of what's at stake: the health of the Earth that sustains us. When we ground ourselves, we ground our perspectives, reminding ourselves of the importance of environmental sustainability. This, in turn, can inspire us to take actionable steps towards protecting the environment, from reducing waste and conserving water to advocating for environmental policies and educating others about sustainable practices.

Concluding Thoughts

Grounding, in essence, encourages a return to nature, fostering a deep, physical connection with the Earth that can inspire a sense of responsibility towards our environment. It reminds us of our intrinsic link to the natural world and the importance of preserving it. In an era marked by environmental challenges, grounding provides a pathway towards increased environmental awareness, promoting sustainable actions for the health of our planet and future generations. By engaging in grounding, we do not just stand on the Earth; we stand with it.

Grounding and Environmental Sustainability

Discussing how Grounding practices can foster a deeper connection with nature and promote environmental awareness.

In today's fast-paced, highly digital world, it's easy to feel distanced from nature. Modern life can be highly disconnecting, encouraging a lifestyle that is removed from the natural world, even though humans have evolved in close contact with nature for thousands of years. In recent times, however, people are becoming increasingly aware of the need to reconnect with nature. This is where grounding, also known as earthing, comes in. Grounding is a practice that promotes a direct connection to the Earth's electrons, fostering a deeper relationship with nature and potentially encouraging environmental sustainability.

Grounding and a Deeper Connection to Nature

Grounding necessitates direct interaction with the natural world. This practice requires us to take the time to stand barefoot on the earth, truly feeling the soil, sand, or grass beneath our feet. It encourages us to slow down, pause, and recognize our intrinsic connection with the world around us. Through the act of grounding, we are physically touching the Earth, reminding us of our relationship with the environment.

This practice can promote a sense of mindfulness, prompting us to take note of the earth beneath our feet, the air around us, and the sky above us. It can make us more aware of the shifts in seasons, the arrival of different wildlife, and the growth of plants and trees. In doing so, grounding can foster a deeper appreciation for the natural world.

Grounding and Environmental Awareness

Beyond promoting personal health benefits, grounding can also play a role in fostering greater environmental awareness. When we regularly make time to connect physically with the Earth, it can make us more cognizant of the changes happening in our environment. It allows us to observe firsthand the effects of different human activities on our surroundings, such as the effects of pollution or the clearing of natural spaces for urban development.

This direct experience can be a potent motivator for increased environmental stewardship. Those who practice grounding might feel a greater sense of responsibility for preserving the environment. They might be more inclined to engage in sustainable practices such as recycling, reducing energy consumption, or advocating for environmental policies.

Grounding as a Path to Sustainable Actions

The act of grounding, in and of itself, is a sustainable practice. It requires no resources other than a patch of natural ground. It doesn't produce waste or use energy. In fact, it serves to remind us of the importance of preserving natural spaces where such grounding activities can take place.

Moreover, grounding can encourage a lifestyle that values simplicity and minimalism. Grounding practices often go hand-in-hand with other natural health practices such as eating a plant-based diet, using natural products, and reducing consumption overall.

Reconnecting with Nature in a Digital Age

In an era dominated by technology, grounding provides a simple and effective way to reconnect with nature. It encourages us to step away from our screens and spend time outdoors. This can foster a greater appreciation for nature, leading to more sustainable behavior.

As we engage in grounding practices, we have an opportunity to reflect on our individual roles within the larger ecosystem. It allows us to contemplate how our daily actions and choices impact the environment. It encourages us to consider how we can make more sustainable choices.

Conclusion

Grounding is a simple practice with potential implications far beyond personal health benefits. It can serve as a tool to foster a deeper connection with nature, promote greater environmental awareness, and encourage more sustainable practices. As we navigate the challenges of the 21st century, grounding offers a path towards a more balanced and sustainable way of life. In reconnecting us to nature, grounding can help us redefine our relationship with the Earth, inspiring us to care more deeply for our shared planet.

7. GROUNDING AND CHILDREN'S HEALTH

Exploring the benefits of Grounding for children's physical and emotional well-being

In a world increasingly dominated by screens and indoor activities, children may often miss out on the simple joys and health benefits of connecting with the natural world. Grounding, also known as earthing, is a practice that may not only improve a child's physical well-being but also enhance their emotional health. Let's explore how grounding can potentially benefit children's health in various ways.

Grounding and Physical Health

Regular physical contact with the Earth can provide children with a range of physical health benefits. Grounding practices are thought to decrease inflammation and pain, improve sleep and relaxation, and boost the immune system, which is particularly beneficial for children as their immune systems are still developing.

Studies have suggested that grounding can help regulate sleep patterns. This may be particularly helpful for children who have difficulty sleeping, reducing night-time awakenings and aiding in a more restful night's sleep. Better sleep can translate to improved concentration, better mood, and higher academic performance.

Grounding and Emotional Well-being

Just as it can benefit adults, grounding can have profound impacts on children's emotional well-being. Spending time outdoors, especially in green spaces, has been shown to reduce stress and anxiety, boost mood, and improve overall mental health in children. Grounding helps children connect with nature, which can instill a sense of calm and tranquility, providing a natural antidote to stress and anxiety.

Engaging in grounding activities can also enhance mindfulness and awareness in children. As they pay attention to the sensations of the Earth beneath their feet, the wind on their skin, or the sounds around them, they can develop a sense of being present in the moment, a skill that can help manage stress and increase overall well-being.

Grounding and Childhood Development

The grounding practice, when made a part of a child's routine, can also contribute to their holistic development. It provides opportunities for exploration, physical activity, and sensorial experiences. Children can improve their motor skills through running barefoot, jumping, or balancing on different surfaces. The different textures, temperatures, and sensations they encounter while grounding can stimulate their senses and promote cognitive development.

Moreover, the grounding practice can foster a sense of independence and confidence as children navigate the natural environment. It also provides ample opportunities for imaginative play, stimulating creativity and cognitive development.

Promoting Grounding in Children

Encouraging grounding in children can be simple and fun. Some effective strategies might include.

Encouraging barefoot play outdoors in safe and suitable environments.

Making grounding a part of your routine, such as a barefoot walk after dinner or grounding playtime.

Encouraging children to sit, lie down or play on the ground, feeling the earth beneath them.

Conclusion

Grounding offers a wealth of potential benefits for children's physical and emotional well-being. As the world becomes increasingly indoor-oriented, grounding offers a way to connect with nature and reap its numerous health benefits. It can be a simple, free, and effective way to boost your child's health and development, grounding them in both a literal and metaphorical sense. Grounding can be a fun way to encourage children to take a break from their screens and spend some time in nature, offering profound benefits for their well-being and development.

8. GROUNDING AND WORKPLACE WELLNESS

Discussing how Grounding practices can be incorporated into the workplace to enhance employee well-being and productivity

In today's fast-paced world, workplaces can be high-stress environments that contribute to physical discomfort, emotional distress, and decreased productivity. Introducing grounding practices into the workplace can offer a fresh perspective and potential solution for fostering well-being and productivity among employees. Let's delve into the concept of grounding, its potential benefits in the workplace, and strategies for integrating it into the corporate environment.

Grounding and Employee Health

Workplace stress can lead to physiological responses such as inflammation, elevated stress hormones, and disturbed sleep. These factors can take a toll on an employee's health over time, leading to decreased immunity, chronic health issues, and burnout. Grounding can potentially counteract these effects.

Research suggests grounding can help reduce inflammation and pain, improve sleep quality, enhance immune response, decrease stress and anxiety, and improve mood. These benefits can contribute to better overall health for employees, reducing sick days and healthcare costs for businesses.

Grounding and Productivity

By reducing stress and improving health, grounding can also impact productivity positively. Employees who are less stressed and enjoy better health are likely to be more engaged and focused, contributing to a more productive and successful business environment.

Furthermore, grounding can also help regulate sleep patterns. Good quality sleep is critical for cognitive functions such as memory, attention, and decision-making. Employees who sleep well are more likely to be alert and productive during their working hours.

Grounding and Employee Engagement

Introducing grounding practices into the workplace can also help foster a sense of community and engagement among employees. Group activities that involve grounding, such as outdoor team-building exercises or wellness retreats, can encourage cooperation and camaraderie among staff. Moreover, these practices signal to employees that their employer cares for their health and well-being, improving job satisfaction and loyalty.

The Benefits of Grounding

To leverage the benefits of grounding in the workplace, businesses can consider several strategies:

Green Spaces: If possible, create green outdoor spaces where employees can take breaks. Walking barefoot on grass or simply sitting in contact with the Earth during breaks can provide grounding benefits.

Walking Meetings: Consider having walking meetings outside, especially for smaller groups or one-on-ones. Employees can walk barefoot if the environment permits.

Team-building Activities: Plan outdoor team-building activities that allow employees to get in touch with the natural environment.

Flexible Breaks: Encourage employees to take short, regular breaks to go outside and connect with the Earth, reducing stress and improving focus.

Educational Workshops: Hold workshops to educate employees about the benefits of grounding and how they can incorporate it into their routines, both at work and at home.

Grounding Mats: For workplaces without access to natural outdoor spaces, grounding or earthing mats can be used. These mats mimic the Earth's natural electrical charge and provide a way to ground indoors.

Conclusion

The introduction of grounding practices into the workplace may offer a novel, cost-effective approach to enhancing employee well-being and productivity. Through creating a more stress-free, health-conscious work environment, businesses can benefit from more engaged, productive, and loyal employees. As we continue to understand the impacts of stress and the benefits of natural therapies like grounding, these practices could become a more common part of the corporate world's approach to employee wellness.

9. GROUNDING AND MINDFULNESS

Exploring the intersection between Grounding and mindfulness practices, and how they can complement each other.

Mindfulness and grounding, often seen as separate practices, can have profound implications for well-being when integrated. Both stemming from holistic paradigms, they promote health, clarity, and tranquility. Let's explore these two concepts, their intersections, and the symbiotic relationship that can enhance their respective benefits.

Understanding Mindfulness

Mindfulness is a form of meditation rooted in Buddhist traditions, now widely used in psychology and wellness practices. It involves focusing one's awareness on the present moment, calmly acknowledging and accepting one's feelings, thoughts, and bodily sensations. Mindfulness practices have been linked to stress reduction, improved mental health, enhanced cognition, and overall improved quality of life.

The Intersection of Grounding and Mindfulness

Grounding and mindfulness, while distinct practices, share fundamental similarities. Both practices bring us into the present moment and foster a connection with our surroundings. They help calm the mind, reduce stress, and enhance physical and emotional well-being. When combined, grounding and mindfulness can complement each other, enhancing the benefits of each.

Present Awareness: Grounding naturally encourages a form of mindfulness. As you feel the grass beneath your feet or the sand between your toes, you're drawn into the present moment. It encourages a mindful awareness of physical sensations, promoting a state of present-centered awareness akin to mindfulness meditation.

Physical Anchoring: Grounding provides a physical connection to the Earth that can be a potent anchor for mindfulness practice. The sensation of the Earth underfoot or the physical connection with the ground can be used as a focus point for mindfulness, helping to keep attention centered in the present moment.

Stress Reduction: Both grounding and mindfulness have been associated with stress reduction. Grounding, through its supposed impact on physiological processes, can reduce inflammation and promote relaxation. Simultaneously, mindfulness aids in managing stress by improving our ability to cope with challenging or stressful situations, reducing anxiety, and improving mood.

Improved Health: Both grounding and mindfulness have been linked to improved health. Grounding may improve sleep, reduce pain, and enhance general well-being. Mindfulness has been associated with improved mental health, better immune response, and even improved cardiovascular health.

Integrating Grounding and Mindfulness

Combining grounding and mindfulness can be a powerful way to enhance physical and emotional well-being. Here's how these two practices can be integrated:

Mindful Grounding Walks: Take a walk barefoot in a safe, natural environment. Pay attention to the sensation of the Earth beneath your feet. Observe any sensations, thoughts, or emotions that arise without judgment.

Grounding Meditation: While grounded, engage in mindfulness meditation. Use the physical sensation of connection with the Earth as an anchor for your attention. When your mind wanders, gently bring it back to the sensation of the Earth beneath you.

Breathing Exercises: While grounded, perform mindful breathing exercises. Breathe deeply and slowly, focusing on each breath's full cycle. Pairing grounding with mindful breathing can enhance relaxation and presence.

In Conclusion

Grounding and mindfulness, two practices steeped in ancient wisdom and increasingly supported by modern science, have the potential to offer significant benefits for mental and physical health. Their integration creates a potent combination that can deepen the experience of presence, enhance relaxation, and foster an improved sense of well-being. As we continue to navigate an often chaotic and stressful world, these practices provide a grounding presence, helping us to live more fully and mindfully in each moment.

10. GROUNDING AND ENERGY MEDICINE

Investigating the relationship between Grounding and other energy-based healing modalities.

The world of holistic health and wellness presents a variety of practices aimed at improving overall well-being and promoting healing from within. Two such practices that have garnered increasing attention are grounding, also known as earthing, and energy medicine. While each practice has its own unique approach, their objectives are aligned in promoting health through natural, energy-based means. This exploration will delve into the realm of grounding and energy medicine, investigating their relationship and potential synergistic effects.

Understanding Grounding

Grounding or earthing is a practice that involves direct contact with the surface of the Earth, such as walking barefoot on grass or sand, sitting or lying directly on the ground, or connecting to the Earth using grounding devices. The premise of grounding is that the Earth's surface is teeming with free electrons, which can be transferred into the body upon direct contact. These electrons are thought to neutralize harmful free radicals in the body, reducing inflammation, improving sleep, reducing stress, and contributing to overall health and vitality.

Understanding Energy Medicine

Energy medicine is a holistic healing approach that involves manipulating the body's energy field to promote health and wellness. This field of therapy encompasses various modalities, including Reiki, acupuncture, Qi Gong, and Healing Touch. The foundational belief in energy medicine is that illness or dis-ease arises when the body's energy flow is disrupted or unbalanced. Energy medicine techniques aim to restore balance to this energy flow, thereby supporting the body's natural ability to heal.

The Interconnection of Grounding and Energy Medicine

Though grounding and energy medicine are different practices, they share a common underlying principle: the harnessing and balancing of energy to promote health and healing. This commonality creates an interesting intersection that allows for the potential integration of these therapies.

Energy Balancing: Both grounding and energy medicine aim to balance the body's energy. Grounding supposedly does so by providing an influx of negatively charged electrons, while energy medicine seeks to balance the body's energy flow through techniques like laying on hands, acupuncture, or energy exercises.

Stress Reduction: Both grounding and energy medicine are associated with stress reduction. Grounding is thought to normalize cortisol levels, thereby reducing stress, while energy medicine often promotes relaxation, which helps alleviate stress and anxiety.

Health Promotion: Both grounding and energy medicine are aimed at promoting overall health. While the specific mechanisms may differ, both practices aim to enhance the body's natural healing capabilities, potentially improving various aspects of health, from sleep to immunity.

Integration of Grounding and Energy Medicine

Given the parallels between grounding and energy medicine, integrating these practices could potentially enhance their respective benefits. Here's how.

Grounding and Energy Medicine Sessions: Practitioners can integrate grounding into energy medicine sessions. For instance, a Reiki session could be conducted outdoors on the Earth's surface, combining the benefits of Reiki's energy balancing with the potential benefits of grounding.

Grounding Practices in Energy Exercises: Certain energy exercises, such as Qi Gong or Tai Chi, could be practiced outdoors while barefoot, incorporating grounding into the energy practice.

Grounding Tools: Grounding tools, such as mats or sheets, could be used in conjunction with energy medicine sessions, providing the grounding effect while energy work is performed.

Conclusion

The world of holistic health continues to bring forward intriguing therapies such as grounding and energy medicine, both aiming to promote wellness by balancing the body's energy. While each stands as a distinct practice, their common objective creates an interesting synergy. The integration of grounding and energy medicine could offer a multifaceted approach to wellness, giving individuals more avenues to explore in their journey to health and well-being. As our understanding of these therapies continues to evolve, it's exciting to consider the potential that lies at the intersection of grounding and energy medicine.

11. GROUNDING AND ENVIRONMENTAL CONSERVATION

Discussing how Grounding practices can promote a deeper connection with the environment and inspire sustainable living.

The age-old practice of grounding or earthing and the more contemporary focus on environmental conservation might seem worlds apart. However, upon closer examination, a profound intersection exists between these two concepts. Both grounding and environmental conservation revolve around our relationship with the natural world, fostering a respect for and understanding of the interconnectedness of life. This exploration will delve into the relationship between grounding and environmental conservation and how this connection might inspire sustainable living.

At its core, grounding is about reestablishing our connection with the Earth, reminding us that we are a part of the natural world. This notion of interconnectedness is crucial for understanding the relationship between grounding and environmental conservation.

Understanding Environmental Conservation

Environmental conservation refers to the protection and preservation of natural resources and ecosystems to prevent their degradation and ensure their continued existence for future generations. The goal of conservation is to maintain the balance of nature, recognizing that every element of an ecosystem is interconnected and interdependent.

This requires a deeper understanding of the impact human actions have on the environment and the development of practices that minimize harm and promote sustainability. These practices can range from recycling and energy conservation at an individual level to policies on deforestation and pollution at a national or global level.

The Interplay of Grounding and Environmental Conservation

The practices of grounding and environmental conservation may be seen as interconnected in multiple ways.

Enhanced Connection to Nature: Grounding literally connects us to the Earth, potentially increasing our appreciation and respect for the natural environment. This deeper connection can inspire more environmentally conscious behavior, as we become more aware of our impact on the Earth.

Awareness of Interconnectedness: Both grounding and environmental conservation promote awareness of the interconnectedness of all life forms. Recognizing this interconnectedness can foster a sense of responsibility to protect and conserve our environment.

Promotion of Health: Grounding is associated with various health benefits, as is living in a clean, sustainable environment. Environmental conservation efforts contribute to better air and water quality, reduced pollution, and preservation of natural spaces, which are crucial for our physical and mental well-being.

Grounding Practices Inspiring Sustainable Living

Grounding, by nature, encourages a more intimate connection with our environment. As we physically connect with the Earth and experience its potential benefits, we might be inspired to adopt more sustainable practices. Here's how:

Nature Appreciation: Regular grounding practices can increase our appreciation for nature, inspiring us to participate in conservation efforts and sustainable practices that protect our natural world.

Mindful Consumption: As grounding promotes mindfulness and awareness, it could potentially influence our consumption habits. Being more conscious of the environmental impact of our choices might inspire more sustainable actions, such as reducing waste, recycling, and choosing environmentally friendly products.

Advocacy and Education: Grounding practitioners, experiencing the benefits of connecting with the Earth, might be motivated to advocate for environmental conservation and educate others about the importance of sustainable living.

Conclusion

Grounding and environmental conservation are intrinsically linked through their focus on our relationship with the natural world. The practice of grounding enhances our connection with the Earth, increasing our awareness of our environment, and potentially inspiring more sustainable practices. As we deepen our understanding of this relationship, we are encouraged to reflect on our roles as stewards of the Earth and consider how our actions impact the environment and our well-being. The synergy of grounding and environmental conservation offers a powerful avenue to promote sustainable living and contribute to the preservation of our precious planet.

12. GROUNDING AND SPIRITUAL GROWTH

Exploring how Grounding practices can support spiritual development and connection.

The practices of grounding, also known as earthing, are fundamentally physical, involving direct contact with the Earth to potentially confer health benefits. However, grounding also has an inherent spiritual aspect, acting as a conduit for enhancing our spiritual growth and connection. This exploration aims to illuminate the relationship between grounding and spiritual development, demonstrating how these practices can profoundly influence our conscious experience and connection to the larger universe.

Grounding: The Physical and Beyond

Grounding is a therapeutic technique that emphasizes reconnecting with the Earth, either through direct skin contact with the Earth's surface or using grounding devices that mimic this connection. Advocates of grounding postulate various health benefits, including reduced inflammation, stress relief, improved sleep, and enhanced energy levels. These effects are proposed to occur due to the transfer of the Earth's free electrons into the body, neutralizing harmful free radicals.

Beyond the physical, grounding also has profound psychological and spiritual implications. It involves experiencing a deep sense of connectedness, not just with the Earth, but with the entire cosmos, reminding us that we are an integral part of the universe.

Spiritual Growth: A Journey Inward

Spiritual growth is an inherently personal journey. It involves expanding one's consciousness, developing a deeper understanding of one's purpose and existence, and cultivating a sense of connectedness with the divine, the universe, or the greater whole, depending on one's belief system.

This journey often involves practices such as meditation, contemplation, mindfulness, and acts of kindness and compassion. It encourages self-awareness, emotional growth, and a deeper understanding of one's values, leading to a more fulfilling and meaningful life.

Grounding and Spiritual Growth: The Connection

At first glance, the physical act of grounding and the intangible concept of spiritual growth might seem unrelated. However, a deeper look reveals a profound connection:

Enhancing Connectedness: Grounding, by its very nature, fosters a deep sense of connectedness with the Earth and the wider universe. This sense of connection is a cornerstone of spiritual growth, facilitating a deeper understanding of our place in the cosmos and our interconnectedness with all life forms.

Promoting Presence and Mindfulness: Grounding techniques often involve being present, focusing on the sensations of the body as it connects with the Earth. This focus on the present moment aligns with mindfulness, a key element of many spiritual practices.

Cultivating Peace and Calm: Grounding is associated with physical relaxation and emotional calm, creating a conducive mental state for spiritual practices such as meditation and contemplation.

Enhancing Self-Awareness: The focus on bodily sensations during grounding can enhance self-awareness, a critical aspect of spiritual growth. Being attuned to our physical presence can serve as a gateway to exploring our deeper, spiritual selves.

The Role of Grounding in Spiritual Practices

Grounding has been incorporated into numerous spiritual practices.

Meditation: Many meditation practices begin with a grounding exercise to center the individual and enhance focus. The sense of connection with the Earth can serve to anchor the mind, facilitating deeper meditative states.

Yoga: Grounding is a crucial component of yoga, which emphasizes the connection between body, mind, and spirit. Grounding poses in yoga help to stabilize and balance the body, fostering a sense of being present and connected.

Energy Work: In various energy healing practices, such as Reiki and Qigong, grounding is vital for maintaining energetic balance and facilitating the flow of energy.

Conclusion

Grounding, in essence, is a powerful tool for spiritual growth. While its physical benefits are increasingly recognized, its spiritual implications offer a unique and profound pathway to self-discovery, connectedness, and expanded consciousness. By promoting presence, self-awareness, and a deep sense of connection, grounding can enhance our spiritual journeys, fostering a more profound understanding of ourselves and our place within the cosmos. Through grounding, we can bridge the physical and spiritual, realizing our integral role in the interconnected tapestry of life and the universe.

13. GROUNDING AND DIGESTIVE HEALTH

The Potential for Therapeutic Connection

The practice of grounding, or earthing, is based on the theory that direct physical contact with the vast supply of electrons on the Earth's surface can have various health benefits. These may range from reducing inflammation and improving sleep quality, to enhancing immune function and even emotional well-being. Among these proposed advantages, one intriguing area of exploration is the potential impact of grounding on digestive health. This exploration will delve into the possible relationship between grounding and digestive disorders, and how this earth connection might play a role in enhancing gut health.

The Significance of Digestive Health

The digestive system is a complex network that plays a crucial role in overall health. It's responsible for breaking down food, absorbing nutrients, and eliminating waste. Moreover, the gut hosts a diverse community of microorganisms, known as the gut microbiota, that contribute to various aspects of health, from nutrient metabolism to immune function and even mental health.

However, when the digestive system is out of balance, it can lead to several health issues, ranging from minor discomforts such as bloating and indigestion to more serious conditions like irritable bowel syndrome (IBS), inflammatory bowel disease (IBD), and gastroesophageal reflux disease (GERD). Hence, maintaining optimal digestive health is essential for overall well-being.

Grounding and Digestive Health: The Connection

Though the scientific exploration of grounding's impact on digestive health is still in its early stages, some mechanisms suggest how grounding might offer benefits:

Reduced Inflammation: Chronic inflammation is a key factor in many digestive disorders, such as IBS and IBD. Grounding has been shown in several studies to reduce inflammation by neutralizing free radicals, potentially aiding in the management of these conditions.

Stress Relief: Stress can significantly impact digestive health, exacerbating symptoms of conditions like IBS and GERD. Grounding has been reported to promote relaxation and reduce stress, potentially helping to alleviate stress-related digestive issues.

Improved Sleep: Poor sleep can adversely affect gut health, contributing to a range of digestive disorders. As grounding has been linked with improved sleep quality, this might indirectly support better digestive health.

Enhanced Immune Response: Our immune system plays a vital role in maintaining gut health, particularly in conditions like IBD where the immune response is dysregulated. Grounding's potential to enhance immune function could, therefore, offer benefits for digestive health.

The Future of Grounding and Digestive Health Research

While these potential mechanisms suggest a promising link between grounding and digestive health, rigorous scientific studies are needed to confirm these effects. Future research could involve randomized controlled trials investigating the impact of grounding on specific digestive disorders or exploring changes in gut microbiota following grounding interventions. Such research could provide valuable insights into the potential of grounding as a natural and accessible tool for enhancing digestive health.

Conclusion

The connection between grounding and digestive health, while intriguing, is still an emerging area of research. Preliminary understandings hint at a potential link, based on grounding's reported benefits of reduced inflammation, stress relief, improved sleep, and enhanced immune response. As our understanding of the complex interplay between environmental factors, lifestyle, and gut health deepens, the practice of grounding might become an important consideration in discussions around maintaining or restoring digestive health. As with all health interventions, individuals should seek professional advice before starting grounding practices, especially those with pre-existing conditions.

14. GROUNDING AND SKIN HEALTH

Discussing the impact of Grounding on skin conditions and overall skin health.

Grounding, also known as earthing, is a therapeutic practice based on the theory that having direct contact with the Earth's surface can be beneficial for our health. This process theoretically allows the body to absorb the Earth's free electrons, promoting a state of physiological equilibrium. Advocates argue that grounding's potential benefits span across various aspects of health, including sleep quality, immune function, and stress reduction. An emerging area of interest is the possible impact of grounding on skin health. This exploration will delve into the potential of grounding as a supportive measure for skin conditions and overall skin health.

Skin Health: A Cornerstone of Overall Well-being

The skin, our body's largest organ, serves multiple vital functions. It provides a barrier against pathogens, regulates body temperature, and enables sensations of touch, heat, and cold. The health of our skin is often a reflection of our overall well-being. However, various factors, such as age, exposure to sun and pollutants, stress, and poor nutrition, can lead to skin issues. These can range from common problems like dryness, acne, and eczema, to more severe conditions like psoriasis and skin cancer. Therefore, exploring all potential avenues, including grounding, for maintaining and enhancing skin health, is of significant interest.

Grounding and Skin Health: The Hypothesized Link

While comprehensive scientific research on grounding's direct impact on skin health is limited, there are several ways grounding could potentially benefit the skin:

Anti-inflammatory Effects: Grounding's potential to reduce inflammation might be beneficial for inflammatory skin conditions like **psoriasis** and **eczema**. Inflammation can lead to skin irritation, redness, and damage. By potentially reducing inflammation, grounding might alleviate these symptoms and support skin healing.

Stress Reduction: Stress is a common trigger for several skin conditions, including **acne** and **psoriasis.** Grounding, being a natural method that promotes relaxation and reduces stress, might indirectly contribute to healthier skin by reducing stress-induced skin flare-ups.

Improved Sleep: Adequate sleep is crucial for skin health as the repair and regeneration of skin cells mainly happen during sleep. Grounding, having been linked to improved sleep quality, could support these restorative processes, promoting overall skin health.

Enhanced Blood Flow: Grounding may improve circulation, thereby enhancing the delivery of oxygen and nutrients to the skin, essential for maintaining skin health and promoting wound healing.

Future Perspectives and Research

Given the potential benefits, it is clear that the area of grounding and skin health warrants further exploration. Future research might focus on conducting rigorous clinical trials to assess the impact of grounding on specific skin conditions. In addition, studies exploring grounding's effect on skin hydration, elasticity, and appearance could be valuable.

Conclusion

While the connection between grounding and skin health is still being understood, initial perspectives suggest a promising link. Given grounding's potential to reduce inflammation, manage stress, enhance sleep, and improve circulation, this practice could be an accessible, natural adjunctive method for supporting skin health. As always, individuals should consult healthcare professionals before starting any new health practices, especially those with existing conditions. Grounding, when used sensibly and as part of a comprehensive skin care routine, may help us maintain our skin's health and vitality.

15. GROUNDING AND HORMONAL BALANCE

Exploring the connection between Grounding and hormonal health.

Grounding, commonly known as earthing, is the practice of physically connecting oneself with the Earth's surface to absorb its naturally occurring free electrons. While this concept might seem unconventional to some, grounding has been a part of numerous ancient traditions, with advocates purporting a range of health benefits. These potential benefits encompass improved sleep, reduced inflammation, enhanced wound healing, and more. An emergent field of interest lies in grounding's possible impact on hormonal health and balance. This comprehensive exploration will delve into the nexus between grounding and hormonal balance, offering insights into this exciting avenue of health research.

Grounding: A Resurgence of Ancient Wisdom

Grounding is based on the theory that direct contact with the Earth's surface, such as walking barefoot on the ground or using specially designed grounding equipment, enables the absorption of free electrons. These electrons may neutralize harmful free radicals in our bodies, fostering a state of physiological balance. The hypothesized benefits, although still a matter of scientific scrutiny, could potentially span various facets of health and well-being.

Hormonal Health: A Delicate Balance

Our hormones, acting as the body's chemical messengers, play an instrumental role in managing virtually every physiological process. From growth and metabolism to mood and reproductive health, the balance of these complex compounds is vital. Disruptions in hormonal balance can lead to a host of health issues, such as **diabetes, thyroid disorders, adrenal fatigue**, and **mood disorders**, to name a few. As such, any practices or interventions that could help support hormonal balance, including grounding, are of considerable interest.

The Grounding-Hormonal Balance Connection: A Hypothesized Mechanism

While the research directly linking grounding with hormonal balance is still evolving, there are several proposed ways that grounding might support hormonal health:

Stress Reduction and Cortisol Regulation: Grounding has been linked to stress reduction, and stress plays a pivotal role in the body's hormonal balance. Chronic stress can lead to the overproduction of cortisol, known as the "stress hormone". This can disrupt the body's hormonal equilibrium, causing an array of health issues. By potentially mitigating stress and promoting relaxation, grounding may support healthier cortisol levels and overall hormonal balance.

Improved Sleep and Melatonin Production: Grounding is hypothesized to improve sleep quality, which is vital for optimal hormonal health. During sleep, the body produces several hormones, including the 'sleep hormone' melatonin. As such, improved sleep quality through grounding could enhance melatonin production and promote overall hormonal balance.

Anti-inflammatory Effects: Chronic inflammation can negatively impact the endocrine system, leading to hormonal imbalances. By potentially reducing inflammation, grounding could indirectly support healthier hormonal function.

Future Research and Perspectives

While the potential benefits of grounding on hormonal health are promising, more rigorous scientific research is required to solidify this connection. Well-designed clinical trials evaluating grounding's impact on specific hormonal conditions and levels could be valuable. Furthermore, research could investigate the use of grounding as a complementary therapy alongside traditional treatments for hormonal imbalances.

Conclusion

Grounding, with its potential for stress reduction, sleep improvement, and anti-inflammatory effects, holds promise for supporting hormonal balance. As our understanding of the grounding-hormonal balance nexus evolves, it could offer valuable insights for preventive health, disease management, and holistic well-being. However, grounding is not a substitute for professional medical advice or treatment. Individuals, especially those with existing hormonal conditions, should always consult with healthcare professionals before integrating new practices like grounding into their routine. Grounding, when practiced responsibly, could potentially be a natural and accessible tool for supporting hormonal health.

16. GROUNDING AND BRAIN HEALTH

Investigating the potential benefits of Grounding for cognitive function and brain health.

Grounding, also known as earthing, is a centuries-old practice that involves coming into direct physical contact with the Earth. This contact could be as simple as walking barefoot on grass, soil, or sand. The premise behind grounding is the idea that the Earth is a natural source of electrons that can help neutralize free radicals in our bodies, and it has been linked with an array of potential health benefits. Recently, the spotlight has turned to the possible effects of grounding on brain health and cognitive function. This exploration delves into the potential connection between grounding and brain health, examining existing research and potential mechanisms behind any benefits.

Brain Health and Cognitive Function: The Cornerstones of Well-being

The brain is our body's command center, regulating countless processes and functions. Maintaining brain health is paramount not just for cognitive function but for overall health and well-being. Cognitive function encompasses abilities **such as memory, attention, perception, learning, problem-solving, and decision-making. Factors such as stress, poor sleep, and chronic inflammation** can negatively impact brain health and cognitive function.

Grounding and Brain Health: Potential Connections

While the body of research specifically exploring the impact of grounding on brain health and cognitive function is currently limited, several hypothesized mechanisms suggest potential benefits:

Stress Reduction and Relaxation: Chronic stress is known to impair cognitive function and brain health. Grounding has been associated with stress reduction and increased relaxation, potentially due to its supposed ability to regulate cortisol, the body's primary stress hormone. By mitigating stress, grounding could indirectly support brain health and cognitive function.

Improved Sleep: Good sleep is essential for brain health, with sleep disturbances linked to cognitive impairments. Grounding is hypothesized to improve sleep quality and duration, potentially supporting brain health and cognitive function.

Reduced Inflammation: Chronic inflammation can harm the brain and cognitive function. By potentially reducing inflammation, grounding may offer indirect benefits to brain health.

Increased Blood Circulation: Grounding is believed to improve blood circulation by reducing blood viscosity. Good circulation is vital for delivering oxygen and nutrients to the brain, supporting optimal function.

Perspectives on Future Research

While the potential mechanisms linking grounding to improved brain health and cognitive function are intriguing, more rigorous and robust research is needed to confirm these hypotheses. Future studies could benefit from employing standardized grounding methods, comprehensive cognitive assessments, and long-term follow-up to examine potential enduring effects.

Conclusion

Grounding presents a potentially natural, accessible, and cost-effective way to support brain health and cognitive function. However, it should be considered as a complementary practice rather than a replacement for traditional medical care. Individuals interested in integrating grounding into their wellness routines should do so responsibly and under the guidance of healthcare professionals. While we wait for more concrete evidence, grounding can be enjoyed for its inherent capacity to reconnect us with nature, promote relaxation, and provide a sense of calm - all of which indirectly contribute to our brain health and cognitive well-being.

17. GROUNDING AND HEART HEALTH

Discussing the impact of Grounding on cardiovascular health and heart disease prevention.

The practice of grounding, also known as earthing, is an age-old method of reconnecting with the earth's natural electric charge. This is typically accomplished by walking barefoot outdoors or using grounding devices that connect to the earth's energy. While grounded, your body can absorb electrons from the earth, which are hypothesized to neutralize harmful free radicals and reduce oxidative stress in the body. Recently, the potential of grounding to affect heart health and aid in preventing heart disease has gained considerable interest. This discussion aims to delve deeper into the impact of grounding on cardiovascular health.

Understanding Grounding and Its Principles

Grounding is predicated on the premise that our planet is a potent source of negative ions. These ions are abundant on the earth's surface, and through direct contact, humans can absorb them. Proponents of grounding suggest that these negatively charged particles can neutralize positively charged free radicals that contribute to inflammation and disease. While grounding has been linked to various health benefits, including reduced inflammation, improved sleep, and lower stress levels, its potential impact on heart health is a topic of emerging interest.

The Heart and Its Importance

The heart is an organ vital to our survival, pumping blood throughout the body to supply necessary oxygen and nutrients. It's a part of our cardiovascular system, which also includes blood vessels and blood itself. Maintaining heart health is critical in preventing cardiovascular diseases such as hypertension, coronary artery disease, and heart failure. These conditions are a leading cause of death globally, making any intervention that might help protect heart health a topic of considerable significance.

Grounding and Heart Health: The Possible Link

There's ongoing research to elucidate the possible impact of grounding on heart health, with several potential mechanisms suggested:

Reduced Inflammation: Chronic inflammation is a known risk factor for heart disease. Grounding has been proposed to reduce inflammation, possibly via neutralization of free radicals, potentially mitigating the risk of cardiovascular diseases.

Stress Relief and Improved Sleep: Chronic stress and poor sleep quality can negatively impact heart health. Grounding, being linked with stress reduction and improved sleep, could thereby indirectly support heart health.

Regulation of Blood Viscosity: Preliminary studies suggest grounding may impact blood viscosity, a critical factor in blood circulation and heart health. Decreased blood viscosity could improve circulation, reducing the workload on the heart.

Moving Forward: The Need for More Research

While these hypotheses provide a compelling argument for grounding's potential benefits for heart health, they are yet to be confirmed by robust, large-scale research. As with any scientific claim, it's crucial to have a substantial body of empirical evidence supporting it, gathered through well-designed, rigorous studies. Grounding, while promising, requires further exploration to understand its full effects on the heart and cardiovascular system. It's crucial that any claims about its benefits are based on comprehensive, peer-reviewed research.

Conclusion

The practice of grounding, with its potential anti-inflammatory and stress-reducing effects, may well have a place in a holistic approach to heart health. However, it should not be seen as a replacement for traditional medical care or proven heart-healthy practices such as regular exercise, a balanced diet, and not smoking. As always, it is recommended to discuss any new health practice with a healthcare provider to ensure it is safe and suitable for individual circumstances. Meanwhile, as we await further research, grounding can be enjoyed for its ability to reconnect us with nature and promote overall well-being. The practice offers a chance to pause, unwind, and attune to the natural rhythms of the earth—a respite that in itself may have profound benefits for our heart health.

18. GROUNDING AND ENVIRONMENTAL JUSTICE

Exploring how Grounding practices can promote equitable access to nature and environmental resources.

Grounding, also known as earthing, is a practice that involves direct skin contact with the surface of the earth. It's a simple act with potential benefits ranging from reducing inflammation to promoting better sleep. While these potential health benefits are important, grounding is also tied to a larger socio-environmental issue: environmental justice. This concept involves fair treatment and meaningful involvement of all people, regardless of race, color, national origin, or income, in the development, implementation, and enforcement of environmental laws, regulations, and policies. In essence, environmental justice is about ensuring equitable access to environmental resources and benefits, like clean air, water, and the earth itself. Grounding, as a practice, can promote this access, and contribute to the broader discourse on environmental justice.

Grounding: A Tool for Environmental Awareness and Connection

The process of grounding necessitates direct interaction with the natural environment, fostering a direct, sensory connection with the earth. This connection can foster a deeper appreciation of the environment and its importance to our health and well-being. As we engage more with the natural world, we're more likely to care about its preservation and advocate for its protection. In this way, grounding can contribute to raising environmental awareness and promoting behaviors that respect and preserve our natural surroundings.

Environmental Justice: An Overview

Environmental justice is an important facet of broader social justice concerns. It involves striving for equal distribution of environmental benefits, like access to natural spaces, and burdens, like exposure to pollution, among all communities. Historically, marginalized and poor communities have often borne the brunt of environmental hazards, while also having limited access to environmental benefits. These communities often lack green spaces for recreation and grounding, leading to disparities in health outcomes and quality of life.

The Intersection of Grounding and Environmental Justice

Grounding can play a role in the pursuit of environmental justice in several ways.

Promoting Equitable Access to Green Spaces: Grounding underscores the importance of having access to clean, natural spaces. By highlighting the potential health benefits of such access, grounding can drive efforts to create more green spaces in urban environments and protect existing natural spaces.

Building Community Connection: Grounding practices, when performed as a group, can help build community connections. It can create a common goal - preserving and enhancing local natural spaces, which can drive local environmental justice initiatives.

Empowering Individual Action: Grounding offers individuals a simple and direct way to interact positively with the environment. Each time a person chooses to ground, they demonstrate the value of nature for personal well-being. This personal connection can spur individuals to advocate for environmental justice in their communities.

Fostering Holistic Health Approaches: Grounding can be part of a holistic approach to health that includes access to clean air, water, and soil. Promoting grounding can draw attention to the importance of these basic environmental necessities, pushing for policies that ensure their equitable distribution.

Challenges and Considerations

While grounding has the potential to promote environmental justice, there are challenges to consider. Not everyone has safe access to natural spaces for grounding, and simply advocating for grounding without addressing this access issue could exacerbate health disparities. Additionally, it's important to remember that while grounding may contribute to environmental justice, it's not a solution in itself. Addressing environmental justice requires structural changes, policy reforms, and collective action.

Conclusion

Grounding, while a personal practice, has implications for broader social and environmental issues. By promoting a direct, tangible connection to the earth, grounding can highlight the importance of equitable access to natural spaces, contributing to the larger discourse on environmental justice. As we ground ourselves, we can also ground our commitment to a fairer, more equitable world, where everyone has the opportunity to connect with and benefit from our shared environment.

19. GROUNDING AND THE GUT-BRAIN AXIS

Investigating the relationship between Grounding and the gut-brain connection.

Grounding, or earthing, is an age-old practice that has been rekindled in the modern world due to the host of potential health benefits it may offer. This practice involves coming into direct skin contact with the earth's surface, thus establishing a physical connection that facilitates the transfer of electrons from the earth to the body. These electrons act as natural antioxidants, fighting inflammation, boosting immunity, and promoting general well-being. However, there's an intriguing area of grounding's effects that is still relatively unexplored: its influence on the gut-brain axis.

Understanding the Gut-Brain Axis

The gut-brain axis is a bidirectional communication system between our central nervous system (brain and spinal cord) and our gut or digestive tract. This system allows the brain to send signals to the gut and vice versa. It includes direct pathways through the nervous system, as well as indirect routes through the immune system and hormones.

Moreover, this connection is deeply intertwined with the gut **microbiome**, the trillions of **microorganisms** residing in our gut. These **microbiotas** play a crucial role in our health, influencing everything from digestion to mental health. Disruptions in this microbial ecosystem can affect the gut-brain axis and contribute to various health issues, including mental health disorders, **neurodegenerative diseases**, and **gastrointestinal** conditions.

Grounding and the Gut-Brain Axis: A Possible Connection

The relationship between grounding and the gut-brain axis may seem far-fetched at first glance. However, considering the broad benefits of grounding and the extensive influence of the gut-brain axis on our health, it's plausible that a connection exists. Here's how grounding might interact with the gut-brain axis:

Reduced Inflammation: Grounding is known for its potential to reduce inflammation. Inflammatory processes in the gut can disrupt the balance of gut microbiota and negatively affect the gut-brain axis. By combating inflammation, grounding might help maintain gut health and, by extension, support a healthy gut-brain connection.

Stress Reduction: Grounding has been associated with stress reduction. High stress levels can harm gut health by altering the gut microbiota and increasing gut permeability, which can lead to inflammation and other issues. These changes can subsequently impact the gut-brain axis. By reducing stress, grounding could indirectly support gut and brain health.

Improved Sleep and Circadian Rhythms: Grounding may help regulate sleep and circadian rhythms. Disturbances in these areas have been linked to gut microbiome alterations and gut-brain axis dysfunction. Therefore, grounding's potential positive impact on sleep and circadian rhythms could translate into benefits for the gut-brain axis.

Research and Future Directions

The possible relationship between grounding and the gut-brain axis remains largely unexplored, and much of the above is speculative based on our current understanding of grounding and the gut-brain axis separately. Rigorous scientific research is needed to understand if, how, and to what extent grounding influences the gut-brain axis.

Such research could encompass studies examining changes in gut microbiota following grounding interventions, investigations into the impact of grounding on gut-related conditions, and trials exploring how grounding affects mental health conditions linked to the gut-brain axis.

In Conclusion

The possible link between grounding and the gut-brain axis presents an exciting frontier in grounding research. As we deepen our understanding of both the gut-brain axis and grounding, we may uncover new dimensions of how grounding contributes to our health and well-being. And who knows? Maybe in the future, we'll have a whole new perspective on the phrase "getting back to our roots" – where it's not just about reconnecting with the earth, but also fostering the essential connection between our gut and brain.

20. GROUNDING AND SOCIAL CONNECTION

Discussing how Grounding practices can foster a sense of connection and community.

The art and science of grounding, often referred to as earthing, involves the formation of a direct physical connection between our bodies and the Earth's surface. Walking barefoot on the grass, sand, or soil, gardening without gloves, or any other activity that brings our skin into contact with the ground helps us establish this bond. The benefits of this simple, age-old practice have been explored extensively in the context of physical health, demonstrating a reduction in inflammation, improved sleep, enhanced wound healing, and more. Yet, one of the often-overlooked aspects of grounding is its potential to foster social connection and community building. This exploration brings together the cultural, psychological, and physiological dimensions of grounding as they relate to social connection.

The Social Nature of Grounding Practices

Grounding practices often involve activities that encourage shared experiences. For instance, group yoga or meditation sessions in parks, community gardening projects, or simple shared experiences of walking barefoot on a beach or in a park. These shared experiences provide an opportunity to connect with others, fostering a sense of community and belonging. They create a common ground — literally and metaphorically — for people to come together, irrespective of their backgrounds, beliefs, or lifestyle.

Psychological Aspects of Grounding and Social Connection

The psychological impacts of grounding may also contribute to improved social connection. Grounding can help reduce stress and anxiety, enhance mood, and improve sleep—factors that are closely linked to our social behavior and interpersonal relationships. By improving our overall psychological wellbeing, grounding can make us more open to social interactions and deepen our relationships with others.

Moreover, grounding can foster a heightened sense of awareness and mindfulness. Being mindful can improve our social skills, like active listening and empathy, as it encourages us to be present in the moment and attuned to ourselves and others.

Cultural Implications of Grounding and Community Building

Many indigenous cultures and ancient civilizations understood the profound connection between humans and the Earth. For them, grounding was not just a physical act but also a spiritual practice that fostered a sense of community.

Even in modern times, grounding practices can serve as a bridge, connecting individuals from various cultural backgrounds. Whether it's a group of city dwellers attending a grounding retreat or a multicultural gathering at a local park, grounding practices provide opportunities for cultural exchange and learning, thereby strengthening social bonds and community spirit.

Physiological Connections Between Grounding and Social Well-being

Grounding influences various physiological processes, some of which are indirectly related to social connection. For instance, grounding has been associated with the regulation of cortisol, a hormone related to stress and anxiety. Lower cortisol levels can lead to a state of relaxation and openness, favoring social engagement and connection.

Furthermore, the physical health benefits of grounding, such as improved sleep and reduced inflammation, can also have a ripple effect on our social lives. Feeling physically well often equates to having more energy and willingness to engage in social activities.

Future Research Directions and Conclusion

Though there are plausible links between grounding and social connection, it's important to acknowledge that this is an emerging field. There's a need for more rigorous scientific studies to understand the mechanisms and extent of these associations better.

Research could involve controlled experiments on the impacts of grounding activities on group cohesion and community feeling, or longitudinal studies to assess the long-term effects of regular grounding on social relationships.

The exploration of grounding's impact on social connection reminds us that we are not isolated beings. As we ground ourselves, we don't just connect with the Earth—we also create opportunities to connect with others. In a world that's increasingly digital and often disconnected, grounding practices may offer a way back to our roots and toward each other. In the end, grounding might not only be about reconnecting us to the Earth, but also about fostering our innate need for social connection and community.

21. GROUNDING AND THE POWER OF VISUALIZATION

Exploring how visualization techniques can enhance the Grounding experience.

The practice of grounding, also known as earthing, connects us to the Earth, fostering physical wellness and inner calm. This simple act of coming into direct contact with the Earth's surface — be it walking barefoot on the grass, swimming in the sea, or just sitting on the ground — can yield profound health benefits. When combined with the power of visualization, a psychological technique involving the use of mental imagery, the grounding experience can be greatly enhanced. This exploration delves into the interplay between grounding and visualization and how these twin techniques can deepen our connection with the Earth and ourselves.

Visualization: A Powerful Mental Tool

Visualization, as a technique, involves creating a mental image or intention of what you desire to happen or feel. By constructing vivid mental pictures, one can 'fool' the mind into believing that the visualized scenario is real, leading to physiological responses and changes. This technique has been used extensively in various fields, from sports psychology where athletes visualize successful performances, to health and wellness spaces where individuals visualize healing processes.

The Synergy of Grounding and Visualization

Integrating visualization with grounding can create a powerful synergy, enhancing the effectiveness of the grounding practice and providing a deeper, more immersive experience. When grounding, visualization can be used to heighten the sense of connection with the Earth. One common visualization technique involves imagining roots growing from one's body into the ground, a symbolic representation of becoming one with the Earth.

Enhanced Physical Health through Visualization and Grounding

Grounding, by itself, has been shown to reduce inflammation, improve sleep, and enhance wound healing, among other benefits. When combined with visualization, these benefits could be amplified. Visualizing the body healing or visualizing the transfer of energy between oneself and the Earth during grounding could potentially boost the immune system, expedite healing processes, and foster overall physical well-being.

Cultivating Mental Wellness with Grounding and Visualization

Grounding and visualization also have immense potential in promoting mental wellness. Grounding helps reduce stress and anxiety and improve mood. Visualization can complement these effects by fostering positive mental states. For instance, visualizing peaceful and serene Earth-related images during grounding can augment feelings of tranquility and inner peace. This combination can prove particularly useful in managing conditions like stress, anxiety, and depression.

Connecting with the Earth on a Deeper Level

Beyond physical and mental health benefits, the combination of grounding and visualization can deepen our relationship with the Earth. Visualizing oneself as an integral part of the Earth ecosystem during grounding can foster a sense of belonging and interconnectedness, which can be both comforting and inspiring. This connection can promote a greater appreciation for nature and drive individuals towards more sustainable practices.

Future Directions and Conclusion

While the intersection of grounding and visualization offers promising potential, more research is required to understand this synergy better. Future studies could focus on quantifying the additive effects of visualization in grounding practices and deciphering the specific mechanisms at play.

In conclusion, the combination of grounding and visualization offers a holistic wellness approach, enhancing our physical health, promoting mental tranquility, and deepening our connection with the Earth. This fusion of practices presents a path towards a balanced and harmonious existence, tuned in with our inner selves and the world around us. As we ground ourselves and visualize our connection with the Earth, we become more rooted — not just in the soil, but within our very essence.

22. GROUNDING AND THE POWER OF AFFIRMATIONS

Investigating how affirmations can amplify the benefits of Grounding.

Grounding, also known as earthing, is a practice that connects us to the Earth's surface, and it has been linked to numerous health benefits, such as reduced inflammation, improved sleep, and better mood regulation. When combined with the power of affirmations — positive, empowering statements about oneself or one's situation — grounding can become an even more potent tool for enhancing health and wellbeing. This exploration delves into the symbiotic relationship between grounding and affirmations, illuminating how the deliberate use of positive self-talk can bolster the efficacy of grounding.

Affirmations: The Power of Positive Self-Talk

Affirmations involve consciously choosing words that will either help eliminate something from your life or create something new in your life. They're brief, powerful statements that, when you say or think them, become the thoughts that create your reality. These statements are typically present-tense and oriented towards the positive, providing a mental image of the state one wishes to achieve.

Affirmations have found a firm place in psychology and self-help paradigms, heralded for their capacity to alter our mental landscape, engender positive emotions, and even change behaviors. They function by influencing our subconscious mind, facilitating a shift in thinking patterns and perceptions.

The Interplay of Grounding and Affirmations

The act of grounding can be augmented by the use of affirmations. As grounding aligns our physiological rhythms with the Earth's, affirmations can assist in aligning our mental and emotional state with our desired outcomes. When you're grounding, the act of consciously focusing your mind on positive affirmations can provide a twofold benefit. Firstly, it can help quieten the mind, easing stress and anxiety, and secondly, it can foster a stronger sense of purpose and positivity.

Physical Wellness through Grounding and Affirmations

Grounding impacts several physical parameters, from reducing chronic pain to enhancing wound healing. When we introduce affirmations to the mix, these benefits can be enhanced. For instance, during grounding, using affirmations like "My body is healing and regenerating" can instill a positive mindset and, through the mind-body connection, potentially aid the healing process.

Boosting Mental Wellbeing with Grounding and Affirmations

Grounding and affirmations have a significant role in fostering mental wellbeing. Grounding helps center us, reducing stress and anxiety. Simultaneously, affirmations can reinforce our mental resilience and self-efficacy. Combining these two can result in a potent antidote to stress, anxiety, and negative thinking patterns. For example, grounding in nature while repeating affirmations such as "I am calm and centered" can help create a relaxed mental state.

Building a Deeper Earth Connection

The combination of grounding and affirmations can facilitate a more profound, mindful connection with the Earth. Affirmations centered on one's relationship with nature and the Earth, such as "I am one with nature" or "The energy of the Earth nourishes me," can foster a sense of belonging and interconnectedness that amplifies the grounding experience.

Future Research and Conclusions

While the integrative use of grounding and affirmations seems promising, scientific research exploring this combination is needed. Future studies could focus on measuring the additive or synergistic benefits of these practices on both physical and mental health outcomes.

In conclusion, the alliance of grounding and affirmations offers an effective strategy for holistic health, nurturing our physical wellbeing, promoting mental resilience, and deepening our bond with the Earth. As we tune into the Earth's rhythm and tap into the power of positive self-talk, we harness an invaluable tool for healing, personal growth, and fostering a greater appreciation of our planet.

23. GROUNDING AND THE POWER OF CRYSTALS

Discussing how crystals can be used in conjunction with Grounding practices to enhance energy and intention.

Grounding, or earthing, is the practice that involves making a direct physical connection with the Earth, and has been touted for its ability to foster numerous health benefits, including reducing inflammation, improving sleep quality, and promoting emotional wellbeing. Alongside grounding, the use of crystals in healing practices has been a prevalent phenomenon across various cultures and ages. The purported power of crystals lies in their ability to hold and emit energy vibrations, and each **crystal** type is believed to have specific vibrational properties and healing attributes. This exploration unpacks the complementary relationship between grounding and crystals, investigating how these tangible elements of the Earth can be utilized together to amplify energy and intention.

Understanding the Essence of Crystals

Crystals are solid materials, whose atoms are arranged in a highly ordered, repeating pattern extending in all three spatial dimensions. These natural substances are formed over thousands, if not millions of years, through processes such as magma cooling or the evaporation of water, and their formation is a testament to the Earth's capacity for creation and transformation. The healing properties of crystals are believed to stem from their inherent vibrational frequencies, which can interact with the body's energy field, or aura.

Integrating Crystals into Grounding Practices

The integration of crystals into grounding practices can be seen as a natural synergy since both grounding and crystals represent tangible connections to the Earth. During grounding, holding or being in proximity to certain crystals can potentially amplify the energetic impact of the practice. Crystals can be selected based on their specific properties that align with one's healing intentions.

Physical Wellness and Crystal-enhanced Grounding

When grounding is used for physical wellness, such as pain reduction or enhancing sleep, crystals associated with these properties can be incorporated. For instance, **amethyst is often used for its purported ability to improve sleep quality**, and **clear quartz is believed to enhance overall energy and vitality.** Using these crystals during grounding could potentially enhance these physical benefits.

Mental and Emotional Wellness through Crystal-enhanced Grounding

Crystals have long been utilized for mental and emotional healing. Rose quartz, for example, is associated with heart healing and promoting feelings of love and compassion. Lapis lazuli is often used for boosting mental clarity and promoting truthful communication. When grounding for mental or emotional wellness, using these crystals could potentially amplify the grounding effect.

Earth Connection and Crystal-enhanced Grounding

The use of crystals can foster a deeper connection to the Earth. Each crystal, formed within the Earth's crust, carries an imprint of the Earth's transformative power and life-sustaining energy. During grounding, using crystals can serve as a reminder of this profound Earth connection and encourage a sense of awe and gratitude for the planet.

Future Research and Conclusions

While the incorporation of crystals into grounding practices holds potential, more scientific research exploring this combination is necessary. Future studies could look into measuring the possible enhanced benefits of grounding with crystals on both physical and mental health outcomes.

In conclusion, the combination of grounding and crystals offers a unique way to connect with the Earth's energy. Each practice, alone, provides a means of balancing the body's energy and promoting wellbeing. Together, they could potentially offer a complementary method for grounding one's energy, setting clear intentions, and fostering a profound sense of Earthly connection. Harnessing the Earth's power in this tangible way can serve as a potent reminder of our intrinsic connection to the planet, facilitating both personal wellness and a greater sense of planetary stewardship.

24. GROUNDING AND THE POWER OF BREATHWORK

Deepening the Earthing Experience through Conscious Breathing.

Grounding, or earthing, is the practice of connecting the human body directly to the Earth's surface energy. This natural method of charging the body with the Earth's electrons has been associated with numerous health benefits, including reducing inflammation, promoting sleep, and balancing the body's circadian rhythms. Complementary to grounding, breathwork, the conscious control of breathing patterns, is another tool utilized in personal development and holistic health disciplines. It aids in influencing mental, emotional, and physical states. This discussion explores how breathwork techniques can enhance and deepen the grounding experience.

Breathwork: An Overview

Breathwork, a broad term encompassing various breathing techniques, is used in many disciplines to create consciousness and connectivity within the self. Techniques range from calming practices, like deep belly breathing or four-square breathing, to more vigorous and stimulating methods, like the Wim Hof Method or Holotropic Breathwork. These conscious breathing practices have been demonstrated to influence the autonomic nervous system, stress responses, emotional well-being, and overall health.

Integrating Breathwork and Grounding

Breathwork and grounding are harmonious practices, as they both involve natural, accessible tools (breath and the Earth), and are recognized for their stress-reducing, healing, and wellness-enhancing properties. By combining the two, one can potentially experience a deeper level of mindfulness, presence, and connection to the Earth.

Enhancing Physical Well-being through Breathwork and Grounding

Grounding can help reduce inflammation and promote healing by restoring the body's natural electrical balance. Concurrently, breathwork practices, like deep, diaphragmatic breathing, can stimulate the parasympathetic nervous system, fostering relaxation and aiding in stress reduction. The act of mindful breathing while grounding may enhance these benefits, promoting a greater sense of physical calm and well-being.

Deepening Emotional and Mental Well-being with Breathwork and Grounding

Grounding helps to stabilize mood and regulate stress hormones, potentially reducing symptoms of anxiety and depression. Similarly, certain breathwork techniques are recognized for their ability to support emotional processing and mental clarity. By focusing on conscious breath control during grounding, one may achieve a deeper sense of mental calm, emotional balance, and mindfulness.

Promoting Earth Connection through Breathwork and Grounding

Both grounding and breathwork foster a profound connection to nature and life's basic processes. Through grounding, we connect physically to the Earth, while breathwork helps us connect to the life-sustaining process of respiration, a reminder of the interconnectivity of all living beings. Utilizing breathwork during grounding practices can deepen this sense of connection and enhance a feeling of belonging to the Earth and its cyclical rhythms.

Future Directions and Conclusions

While anecdotal evidence and preliminary research suggest potential benefits from combining breathwork and grounding, more rigorous scientific studies are needed to explore this symbiotic relationship. Future research might consider investigating physiological markers, such as heart rate variability, stress hormone levels, and immune response, to measure the potential enhanced benefits of combined grounding and breathwork practices.

In conclusion, integrating breathwork with grounding offers an accessible, natural method to potentially enhance overall well-being. The combination could support a deeper state of relaxation, promote emotional balance, and foster a profound sense of connection with our planet. This symbiotic approach represents a promising avenue for future exploration in the field of holistic health, further enriching our understanding of the powerful connection between our bodies and the Earth.

25. GROUNDING AND THE POWER OF YOGA

Grounding and the Power of Yoga: Investigating the Integration of Grounding Practices into Yoga Routines for Enhanced Mind-Body Connection.

Grounding or earthing is the therapeutic practice of making direct contact with the earth's surface to absorb its beneficial electrons. The concept is rooted in the understanding that our planet's surface possesses a limitless and continuously renewed supply of free electrons, which have natural antioxidant effects. Yoga, on the other hand, is an ancient discipline involving a series of physical postures, breath control, and meditation that aims to integrate the mind, body, and spirit. This discourse explores how integrating grounding practices into yoga routines can enhance the overall mind-body connection, potentially augmenting yoga's established benefits.

Understanding Yoga: Philosophy and Practice

Yoga is a mind-body practice that originated in ancient India. It is a comprehensive discipline that combines physical postures (asanas), breath control (pranayama), and meditation (dhyana) to foster physical strength, relaxation, and mental clarity. Yoga is recognized for various health benefits, such as increased flexibility and muscle strength, enhanced respiratory and cardiovascular function, balanced metabolism, and improved athletic performance. Moreover, it supports mental well-being by reducing stress, promoting relaxation, and enhancing body awareness.

Grounding and Its Health Benefits

Grounding or earthing refers to making direct contact with the earth, such as walking barefoot on the grass, swimming in natural bodies of water, or using conductive systems that transfer the earth's electrons to the body. This practice is believed to counteract the harmful effects of free radicals in the body, promoting various health benefits. These include reducing inflammation, improving sleep quality, reducing stress and anxiety, enhancing immune function, and supporting overall well-being.

Integration of Grounding and Yoga

The combination of grounding and yoga can be a synergistic practice that harnesses the benefits of both modalities. By practicing yoga asanas outdoors in direct contact with the earth, one can enhance the grounding effect, making the practice more potent and restorative. This connection can add another dimension to yoga practice, deepening the sense of being present and connected to the natural world, potentially enhancing its physical and mental benefits.

Enhancing Physical Well-being through Grounding and Yoga

The integration of grounding and yoga could amplify the physical benefits of both practices. Yoga improves strength, flexibility, and balance, while grounding reduces inflammation and boosts recovery. The combined practice can potentially offer enhanced physical well-being, aiding in injury prevention, promoting faster recovery, and supporting overall fitness and health.

Deepening Mental and Emotional Well-being with Grounding and Yoga

Yoga is well-known for promoting mental clarity, reducing stress, and supporting emotional balance. Simultaneously, grounding has been linked to improved sleep, reduced stress, and mood regulation. Practicing yoga while grounded could potentially deepen these mental and emotional benefits, fostering a more profound sense of calm, balance, and inner peace.

Promoting Earth Connection through Grounding and Yoga

Both grounding and yoga foster a sense of connection – grounding to the earth, and yoga to the self. Practicing yoga while grounded can enhance this sense of connectedness, creating a unique opportunity to feel more in tune with the natural world, enhancing environmental awareness and fostering a profound sense of belonging.

Potential Challenges and Future Directions

While integrating grounding and yoga seems beneficial, it might not always be feasible, given environmental constraints or weather conditions. To overcome this, grounding mats or grounding yoga mats can be used. These tools, when connected to a grounding wire in the home, can help simulate the effects of direct contact with the earth.

Future research should focus on exploring the potential amplified benefits of combining grounding and yoga, assessing both qualitative (self-reporting of stress, well-being, etc.) and quantitative (biomarkers such as cortisol levels, inflammatory markers, etc.) measures.

In conclusion, the integration of grounding practices into yoga routines holds the potential to enhance the overall mind-body connection, harnessing the physical and mental benefits of both practices. This synergy can provide a deeper state of relaxation, enhanced physical well-being, and a heightened sense of connection with the earth, making it a promising area for future exploration in holistic health and wellness practices.

26. GROUNDING AND THE POWER OF MEDITATION

Discussing How Grounding Practices Can Deepen Meditation Experiences and Promote Inner Peace.

Grounding, also known as earthing, is a practice that involves making direct contact with the Earth's surface. By walking barefoot on grass or soil, swimming in natural bodies of water, or utilizing grounding equipment, we can absorb the Earth's beneficial electrons. These electrons have natural antioxidant effects, contributing to numerous health benefits such as reduced inflammation, improved sleep quality, and decreased stress levels.

Meditation, a mindfulness practice that dates back thousands of years, has been praised for its ability to bring inner peace, reduce stress, increase self-awareness, and promote emotional health. This discourse aims to investigate how combining grounding practices with meditation can deepen the meditative experience and further contribute to overall wellbeing and inner peace.

Understanding Meditation: The Journey Within

Meditation is a mental discipline wherein one aims to go beyond the reflexive thinking mind into a deeper state of relaxation or awareness. There are countless ways to meditate, but the objective is usually the same – to bring tranquility and clarity to the mind. Meditation practices can range from focusing on one's breath or a specific thought to movement-based techniques such as Tai Chi or Yoga.

These practices have proven to have profound impacts on an individual's health and wellness. Not only does meditation help reduce stress and anxiety, but it also has the potential to improve concentration, increase self-awareness, and promote a positive outlook on life.

Combining Grounding and Meditation

Merging the grounding and meditation practices may offer synergistic benefits, deepening the overall meditative experience. Grounding can serve as a facilitator for meditation, creating an environment conducive to relaxation and improved focus. It offers a physical connection to nature, which can help still the mind and foster a sense of inner peace, thereby deepening the meditation practice.

Physiological Benefits of Grounding and Meditation

When meditating while grounded, the physical benefits of both practices can potentially be amplified. Grounding has been shown to normalize the functioning of all body systems, while meditation can lower heart rate and blood pressure and improve breathing. When these practices are combined, the grounding effect can help to further stabilize the body's basic biological rhythms, improve immune response, and reduce inflammation, thereby increasing the benefits of meditation on the physical body.

Psychological and Emotional Benefits of Grounding and Meditation

Psychologically, grounding and meditation can work hand in hand to enhance mental wellbeing. Both practices independently have been shown to reduce stress and anxiety and improve mood. Grounding can help achieve a more tranquil state more quickly during meditation by reducing the effects of electromagnetic fields on the body, and its resulting calming effect can potentially enhance the impact of meditation on mood and anxiety levels.

Enhancing Inner Peace with Grounding and Meditation

Inner peace, often described as a state of mental and spiritual calm, is a common goal of meditation. The physical connection to the Earth provided by grounding can enhance the sense of peace experienced during and after meditation. The combination of both practices can lead to a deeper experience of calm, providing a greater sense of balance and harmony between the mind, body, and the natural world.

Grounding, Meditation, and the Journey to Self-discovery

Grounding and meditation can facilitate self-discovery and self-understanding. Grounding connects us to the earth, while meditation connects us to our inner selves. These combined practices can enhance self-awareness, giving insight into thought processes and emotional responses, and paving the way towards personal growth and self-improvement.

Potential Limitations and Future Directions

While the combination of grounding and meditation shows promise, limitations might include lack of access to natural grounding environments for some people, such as those in urban settings. Grounding technology, such as grounding mats and patches, can be a viable alternative, making grounding more accessible to a broader population.

Further research should be conducted to explore the benefits of combining grounding and meditation practices, including investigating physiological changes and personal experiences of individuals who incorporate these practices into their routine.

In summary, the combination of grounding and meditation presents a unique approach to health and wellbeing. By integrating the physical connection to the Earth with the mental discipline of meditation, individuals may experience deepened meditative states, enhanced wellbeing, and a greater sense of inner peace. These practices present a holistic approach to health that deserves further exploration and recognition.

27. GROUNDING AND THE POWER OF MASSAGE THERAPY

Exploring how Grounding practices can be combined with massage therapy for enhanced relaxation and healing.

Grounding and the Power of Massage Therapy: Exploring How Grounding Practices Can Be Combined with Massage Therapy for Enhanced Relaxation and Healing

Grounding and massage therapy are both practices with ancient roots that promote healing and relaxation. Grounding, or earthing, involves direct physical contact with the earth's surface and its natural electrical charge, which is believed to have numerous health benefits, such as reduced inflammation and improved sleep quality. Massage therapy, on the other hand, uses touch and physical manipulation of the body's soft tissues to relieve tension, promote relaxation, and enhance overall well-being. This discussion aims to explore the potential of integrating these two practices, examining how grounding can complement massage therapy for enhanced relaxation and healing.

Understanding Massage Therapy: The Power of Touch

Massage therapy is a practice that involves manipulation of the body's soft tissues, including muscles, connective tissue, tendons, ligaments, and joints. It is designed to alleviate the discomfort associated with everyday stresses, muscular overuse, and many chronic pain conditions. Massage therapy helps to relax muscle tissue, leading to decreased nerve compression, increased joint space, and range of motion. This can reduce pain and improve function.

The Symbiotic Relationship Between Grounding and Massage Therapy

Grounding and massage therapy may complement each other in a symbiotic relationship, as they both aim for similar outcomes: overall wellness, relaxation, and healing. When these practices are combined, the benefits of each can potentially be enhanced.

For example, grounding before a massage session could prime the body for relaxation, making it more receptive to the therapist's touch. On the other hand, grounding after a massage therapy session could prolong and enhance the therapeutic effects by continuing to reduce inflammation and promote relaxation.

Potential Physiological Benefits of Grounding and Massage Therapy

From a physiological perspective, combining grounding with massage therapy might result in improved outcomes for patients. Both grounding and massage therapy have been found to reduce inflammation and pain. They both also help to relax the body and mind, which can lead to improved sleep, better mood, and overall well-being.

When grounding is added to massage therapy, it can potentially enhance these benefits. For example, the relaxation brought about by grounding may make muscles more pliable and responsive to massage. The antioxidant effects of grounding could also enhance the healing process after a deep tissue massage, reducing post-massage soreness and inflammation.

Psychological and Emotional Benefits of Grounding and Massage Therapy

Grounding and massage therapy also have psychological and emotional benefits. Massage therapy is known to promote relaxation and reduce anxiety, which can be further enhanced by the calming effect of grounding. Grounding itself has been shown to reduce cortisol levels, the primary stress hormone, promoting a state of relaxation and peace.

Combining grounding with massage therapy could provide a comprehensive mind-body relaxation technique that promotes psychological well-being. This could be particularly beneficial for people suffering from stress-related disorders or conditions linked to chronic inflammation.

The Integration of Grounding and Massage Therapy into Wellness Practices

Implementing grounding practices into massage therapy sessions can be simple and practical. This could be as straightforward as conducting massage sessions outdoors in a suitable environment, such as on a beach or in a grassy park, weather permitting. For indoor settings, grounding equipment such as grounding mats or sheets could be utilized.

Potential Limitations and Future Directions

While the integration of grounding and massage therapy holds promise, challenges include access to suitable outdoor spaces for grounding, particularly for urban-dwelling individuals, and the additional cost of grounding equipment for indoor use.

Further research is warranted to explore the potential benefits and synergies of grounding and massage therapy in more detail. Studies could investigate whether grounding indeed enhances the therapeutic effects of massage and the most effective ways of combining these practices.

In conclusion, the combination of grounding and massage therapy may offer a novel approach to promote relaxation and healing. By leveraging the benefits of both practices, this approach could provide a holistic method of enhancing health and well-being. Both practitioners and recipients of massage therapy may find value in incorporating grounding techniques into their routines, possibly leading to enhanced outcomes and an overall more fulfilling experience.

28. GROUNDING AND THE POWER OF SOUND HEALING

Investigating the combination of Grounding practices with sound healing techniques for holistic well-being.

Grounding, also known as earthing, and sound healing are two increasingly popular practices used to promote physical, emotional, and mental well-being. Grounding involves making direct physical contact with the Earth's surface, enabling a transfer of negatively charged free electrons into the body. This is believed to contribute to a host of health benefits. Sound healing, on the other hand, employs various aspects of sound, such as rhythm, frequency, and harmony, to foster healing and well-being. This investigation explores the potential of combining these two therapies as a holistic approach to health and wellness.

Understanding Grounding: The Earthing Connection

Grounding is based on the notion that our bodies are meant to come into contact with the Earth on a regular basis. This contact allows the transfer of free electrons from the Earth's surface into the body, where they act as antioxidants, neutralizing harmful free radicals and potentially reducing inflammation. Grounding has been associated with benefits like reduced stress and anxiety, improved sleep, and enhanced immune function.

Understanding Sound Healing: The Resonance of Health

Sound healing, sometimes referred to as sound therapy, is a practice that employs various aspects of sound to promote healing and well-being. It involves using tools such as musical instruments or the human voice to generate sound vibrations that are perceived not only by the ears but by the entire body. Different frequencies and rhythms can affect the body's functions, potentially easing stress, lowering blood pressure, improving sleep, and reducing pain.

Combining Grounding and Sound Healing: A Symphony of Benefits

The idea of merging grounding and sound healing comes from the recognition that these practices share common therapeutic targets, including stress reduction, promotion of relaxation, and enhancement of overall well-being. Both modalities offer unique pathways to these goals, and their combination may potentially yield synergistic effects, creating an even more powerful holistic healing experience.

For example, a sound healing session can be conducted while the participant is grounded, perhaps sitting or lying on the earth, a beach, or using a grounding mat. The calming and stress-relieving effects of grounding could help the individual become more receptive to the healing properties of the sound therapy. Conversely, the relaxing effect of sound healing could enhance the individual's experience of grounding, leading to a more profound sense of connection with the Earth.

Potential Physiological and Psychological Benefits

Physiologically, the combination of grounding and sound healing may boost the immune system, enhance sleep, and promote self-healing by reducing inflammation and stress hormones in the body. The resulting state of relaxation may also enhance digestion, improve circulation, and stimulate the body's detoxification processes.

Psychologically, both grounding and sound healing are believed to promote a sense of well-being, calm, and relaxation, while reducing anxiety and boosting mood. Combining these practices could provide a comprehensive mind-body relaxation technique, promoting a deeper sense of inner peace, mindfulness, and connection with oneself and the environment.

Challenges and Future Research Directions

Despite the promising potential of combining grounding and sound healing, challenges remain. Access to suitable outdoor locations for grounding is not always possible, particularly for individuals living in densely populated urban environments. Additionally, while the principles of sound healing are generally well-established, the field still faces skepticism from some medical professionals who demand more rigorous scientific evidence to support its efficacy.

Future research should aim to provide rigorous, evidence-based insights into the synergistic effects of grounding and sound healing. Randomized controlled trials could investigate the physiological and psychological effects of these combined practices, shedding light on their potential benefits and limitations.

Concluding Thoughts

The integration of grounding and sound healing presents an exciting frontier in holistic health practices. The merging of these two therapies can offer a unique and powerful tool for promoting health, reducing stress, and enhancing overall well-being. By harnessing the natural power of the Earth's energy and the therapeutic resonance of sound, individuals may discover a profound new pathway to wellness and harmony. This approach underscores the importance of reconnecting with nature and our innate sense of rhythm and harmony, offering a holistic approach to health that can complement conventional medical treatments.

29. GROUNDING AND THE POWER OF HERBAL MEDICINE

Discussing how Grounding practices can be complemented by herbal remedies for overall health and vitality.

The realm of holistic health and wellness has seen the resurgence of many ancient practices, two of which are grounding, often referred to as earthing, and herbal medicine. Grounding, a process of direct physical contact with the Earth's surface, has been observed to offer a myriad of health benefits, including reduced stress and improved sleep. On the other hand, herbal medicine employs plants and their extracts to support the body's natural healing processes. This discussion delves into the intersection of these two practices and how they can be synergistically applied for overall health and vitality.

Understanding Herbal Medicine: The Power of Plants

Herbal medicine, one of the oldest forms of healthcare known to mankind, utilizes plants and plant extracts for therapeutic purposes. Each plant carries unique chemical constituents that can have powerful effects on the human body. Herbal remedies have been used to treat a wide range of ailments, from common colds and digestive issues to chronic diseases such as diabetes and hypertension. They also play a significant role in prevention, supporting immune function, and maintaining overall health.

The Synergy of Grounding and Herbal Medicine: A Pathway to Vitality

Grounding and herbal medicine share an overarching theme of utilizing nature's offerings to promote health and well-being. The combination of these two practices can create a potent synergy for enhancing vitality and overall wellness.

Consider a simple grounding exercise performed outdoors amidst the verdant splendor of a garden. As the body absorbs the Earth's negative electrons, the individual can also inhale the aromatic essences released by the surrounding plants, some of which are known to have therapeutic properties. For instance, the scent of lavender is renowned for its calming effects, while rosemary is known to enhance memory and concentration. Such a holistic experience can contribute to both physiological and psychological wellness.

The incorporation of herbal remedies can also amplify the benefits derived from grounding. For instance, drinking herbal teas made from plants like chamomile or valerian root, known for their calming and sleep-enhancing properties, could potentially enhance the sleep-improving effects of grounding. On the other hand, energizing herbs like ginseng or maca could amplify the invigorating effects of a grounding session.

Potential Benefits and Future Perspectives

Integrating grounding with herbal medicine brings together two potent natural therapies that can complement each other. This combined approach can offer more profound relaxation, enhanced stress relief, improved sleep quality, and overall increased vitality. Moreover, it may also contribute to better immune function, improved digestion, and a more balanced mood, among other benefits.

However, as promising as the combination of grounding and herbal medicine may be, there are still challenges and considerations. Herbal medicine, while generally safe when used correctly, should be administered under the guidance of a qualified healthcare provider, as certain herbs can interact with medications or have side effects.

The call for more research is apparent to provide solid scientific evidence of the synergy between grounding and herbal medicine. Studies could explore the potential additive or synergistic effects of these therapies and offer guidelines for their combined use.

In Conclusion

The marriage of grounding and herbal medicine offers a promising avenue towards enhanced health and vitality. By harnessing the energy of the Earth and the medicinal power of plants, individuals have the opportunity to explore a more holistic approach to wellness that nurtures the body, calms the mind, and soothes the spirit. This integration underscores the importance of reconnecting with nature and recognizing its abundant gifts that can help us maintain and restore our health.

30. GROUNDING AND THE POWER OF REIKI

Exploring the integration of Grounding practices with Reiki energy healing for balance and harmony.

In the contemporary world, ancient healing practices have regained popularity as a counterbalance to the often stressful and disconnected lifestyle of modern societies. Two such practices, grounding and Reiki, have shown immense potential in fostering health, balance, and harmony. This discussion explores the incorporation of grounding, a method of reconnecting with the Earth's energy, with Reiki, a form of energy healing, and how this synergistic combination can contribute to holistic well-being.

Grounding: A Physical Connection to the Earth

Grounding, also known as earthing, is the process of making direct contact with the Earth's surface, such as walking barefoot on the grass or beach. The principle behind grounding is the exchange of electrons between the Earth's surface and our bodies, creating a kind of "electric nutrition," helping to maintain the body's equilibrium, reduce inflammation, and neutralize free radicals.

The benefits of grounding are diverse and impactful. Research has suggested that regular grounding practices can improve sleep, enhance immune function, decrease stress and anxiety, and boost overall vitality.

Reiki: The Universal Life Energy

Reiki, a Japanese technique for stress reduction and relaxation, is often used as a complementary approach in holistic health and wellness. Reiki practitioners use a technique called palm healing or hands-on healing through which a "universal energy" is transferred through the palms of the practitioner to the patient to encourage emotional or physical healing.

Reiki's principles are rooted in the understanding that life energy flows through all living beings. When this energy flow is balanced, one is more capable of being happy and healthy. However, when the life energy is low, individuals are more likely to get sick or feel stressed. Reiki aims to enhance this life energy flow, thereby promoting health and well-being.

Grounding and Reiki: An Energy Synergy for Balance and Harmony

The integration of grounding and Reiki marries two potent energy practices – one anchored in the physical realm (the Earth), and the other rooted in the spiritual realm (universal life energy). This combination may create a powerful synergy for achieving balance and harmony.

Imagine a Reiki session conducted in a natural setting, where the recipient is grounded to the Earth. This situation allows the individual to absorb the Earth's electrons while receiving universal life energy from the Reiki practitioner. This scenario harmonizes the exchange of energies and enhances the overall healing experience.

Integrating grounding with Reiki could amplify the benefits of both practices. Grounding may enhance the energy flow during a Reiki session, allowing the recipient to be more open and receptive to the universal life energy. Simultaneously, Reiki could help channel the Earth's energy absorbed during grounding more effectively throughout the body, thus promoting greater balance and harmony.

Potential Benefits and Considerations

The combination of grounding and Reiki can potentially offer profound health benefits, including improved energy levels, enhanced relaxation, better sleep quality, reduced stress and anxiety, and a stronger sense of overall well-being. This combination may also contribute to a more balanced mood, improved focus and clarity, and deeper spiritual connection.

However, while the integration of these practices is promising, it's important to remember that experiences with grounding and Reiki can vary significantly from person to person. Each individual's receptivity to these practices can be influenced by various factors, such as their overall health, mental state, and openness to energy therapies.

The Path Forward

Despite the potential benefits of combining grounding with Reiki, more research is needed to provide solid evidence of their synergistic effects and to develop guidelines for their integrated use. Future research could also explore whether specific grounding practices are more conducive to Reiki sessions than others, providing practitioners and recipients with valuable insights.

In Conclusion

Uniting the practices of grounding and Reiki presents an exciting opportunity for individuals seeking holistic methods to enhance their health and well-being. The combination of the Earth's energy with universal life energy creates a unique healing synergy that promotes balance, harmony, and overall vitality. The exploration of this integrative approach underscores the value of diverse healing practices and their role in promoting health and well-being in a holistic, interconnected manner.

31. GROUNDING AND THE POWER OF AYURVEDA

Investigating how Grounding practices align with the principles of Ayurveda for optimal health and well-being.

The exploration of holistic health practices often brings together elements of various traditions, marrying ideas and methods that, though originating from different parts of the world, resonate on a similar frequency. Grounding, a practice that encourages connecting physically with the Earth, and Ayurveda, a holistic health system with ancient Indian roots, are two such practices that, despite their different origins, align in their principles and intentions. This essay investigates how grounding practices complement the principles of Ayurveda, offering a combined approach to foster optimal health and well-being.

Grounding: The Energy of the Earth

Grounding, also known as earthing, involves making direct contact with the Earth, typically through barefoot walking or sitting on the ground. The central idea of grounding is the energy exchange that happens when our bodies make contact with the Earth. This transfer of electrons may help reduce inflammation, enhance immune function, improve sleep, and decrease stress levels, providing a host of health benefits grounded in the Earth's natural energy.

Ayurveda: The Science of Life

Ayurveda, often translated as the "science of life," is a holistic system of medicine that originated in India over 5,000 years ago. This comprehensive healing system emphasizes balance in all areas of life, including diet, lifestyle, exercise, sleep, and mental health. It seeks to align the individual's internal rhythms with the natural rhythms of nature, believing that such alignment fosters health and well-being.

Ayurveda is based on the concept of three doshas or life energies: Vata, Pitta, and Kapha, which are combinations of the five fundamental elements of the universe – space, air, fire, water, and earth. According to Ayurveda, health is a state of balance among these doshas, and illness results from an imbalance.

Grounding and Ayurveda: Earth Energy Meets Life Science

The practice of grounding appears to align harmoniously with the principles of Ayurveda. At the most fundamental level, both grounding and Ayurveda emphasize connection with nature as vital for health and well-being. Grounding encourages us to connect physically with the Earth, while Ayurveda motivates us to align our life rhythms with those of nature.

In Ayurvedic principles, each of the doshas corresponds to a combination of the five elements. The element of 'Earth' is present in both Kapha and Vata doshas. Kapha, composed of Earth and Water, governs structure and stability in the body. Grounding, with its Earth-based focus, may particularly benefit those with an excess of Kapha by grounding their energy and stabilizing their bodies. On the other hand, Vata, composed of Space and Air, governs movement and change. Individuals with a predominant Vata constitution, who often struggle with feelings of instability and anxiety, might find grounding practices particularly beneficial, helping them feel more anchored and less anxious.

Potential Benefits and Considerations

The integration of grounding and Ayurveda could potentially offer a wide range of health benefits. These may include improved sleep, reduced inflammation, balanced energy levels, enhanced immune function, and decreased stress and anxiety levels. The alignment of the physical body with the Earth's energy through grounding, coupled with the holistic and personalized approach of Ayurveda, can provide a comprehensive wellness strategy for individuals seeking natural, preventative health measures.

Yet, it's crucial to recognize that Ayurveda is a complex system that requires individualized approaches. While grounding is a universally beneficial practice, Ayurvedic recommendations vary greatly based on one's unique constitution and current state of balance or imbalance. Therefore, integrating grounding with Ayurveda should ideally be guided by a knowledgeable Ayurvedic practitioner.

The Path Forward

The blend of grounding and Ayurveda underscores the potential benefits of integrating diverse health practices. As we continue to validate ancient wisdom with modern science, opportunities for such integrations are likely to increase. Future research could focus on substantiating the beneficial effects of combining these practices and providing practical guidelines for their application.

In Conclusion

In combining grounding with Ayurveda, we invite an intersection of ancient wisdom and contemporary holistic practices that can provide a robust, preventative, and healing approach to health. Aligning the energy transfer from the Earth with the balancing principles of Ayurveda, individuals can harness a potent synergy to foster their overall well-being, proving that sometimes, the best way forward for health is to root ourselves firmly in the natural wisdom of the past.

32. GROUNDING AND THE POWER OF ENERGY PSYCHOLOGY

Discussing how Grounding practices can be combined with energy psychology techniques for emotional healing and transformation.

The landscape of therapeutic modalities in psychology has seen an evolution, blending traditional approaches with newer methods that recognize the interplay between our physical bodies and emotional health. One such area of exploration is energy psychology, a subset of practices that acknowledges and harnesses the body's energy fields to facilitate healing and transformation. Grounding, or earthing, is another practice that delves into the realm of our connection to natural energies, particularly those of the Earth. This article explores the confluence of these two areas — grounding and energy psychology — and discusses how they might combine to foster emotional healing and transformation.

Understanding Grounding

Grounding is a practice that involves making a direct, physical connection with the Earth. This can be achieved through simple acts such as walking barefoot in the grass, sand, sitting or lying directly on the ground. The Earth, as a gigantic electrical object, is continually emitting a field of energy. Grounding proponents posit that direct contact with the Earth allows the body to absorb these beneficial energies, which can promote a wide array of health benefits — ranging from reducing inflammation and improving sleep, to boosting mood and aiding in the recovery from traumatic experiences.

Energy Psychology: An Overview

Energy psychology, on the other hand, is a relatively new branch in the field of psychology. It builds on the principles of traditional psychology, but also integrates elements of ancient spiritual practices and modern quantum physics. Energy psychology posits that our thoughts, behaviors, and emotions are interconnected with our body's energy system. Hence, changes in our energy system can influence our mental, emotional, and physical health.

Techniques in energy psychology often involve tapping on specific points on the body's meridian system (used in acupuncture), visualization, and affirmations. They can be applied to address a range of issues, from anxiety and depression, to phobias, post-traumatic stress disorder (PTSD), and more.

The Intersection of Grounding and Energy Psychology

Grounding and energy psychology intersect in their understanding that energy, in its different forms, significantly influences human health and well-being. They both recognize that an individual's physical, emotional, and mental states are intimately linked with various energy fields—be it the Earth's energy in grounding or the body's meridians in energy psychology.

This convergence offers a platform for integrating grounding and energy psychology for emotional healing and transformation. Grounding, with its focus on connecting with the Earth's energies, can be seen as a tool for centering and stabilizing oneself, creating a calm and receptive state conducive for energy psychology work.

Simultaneously, the practices of energy psychology can guide the directed transformation of emotional states and thought patterns.

Imagine a session that begins with grounding practices to soothe the nervous system and establish a calm, centered state. Once this baseline of calm has been achieved, energy psychology techniques like tapping or psychological kinesiology could be introduced to address specific emotional or psychological issues. This harmonious integration may lead to more effective and sustained therapeutic outcomes.

Potential Benefits and Considerations

The combination of grounding and energy psychology holds promise for offering a more holistic, integrative approach to emotional healing and transformation. By addressing the energy dimensions of our existence along with our physical, emotional, and mental states, these practices can enhance our resilience, deepen self-understanding, and offer powerful tools for coping with stress, trauma, and life's various challenges.

It's essential, however, to remember that while grounding is generally a safe and natural practice for everyone, energy psychology techniques should be employed under the guidance of trained practitioners, particularly when dealing with deep-seated traumas or severe psychological conditions.

The Path Forward

The intersection of grounding and energy psychology marks a significant development in our understanding of holistic health and well-being. However, this is still a growing field, and more scientific research is needed to substantiate the potential benefits of combining these practices. While personal experiences and anecdotal evidence provide some validation, rigorous clinical studies could offer a more comprehensive understanding of the effectiveness of these combined practices.

In Conclusion

The marriage of grounding practices with energy psychology techniques presents a promising frontier for promoting emotional healing and transformation. This integrative approach could offer individuals a powerful and accessible set of tools for managing their emotional health, enhancing resilience, and promoting overall well-being. By harmonizing our connection to the Earth's energies with targeted, therapeutic energy psychology practices, we might discover new paths to healing and self-transformation, honoring the interconnectedness of our body, mind, and the world we inhabit.

33. GROUNDING AND THE POWER OF MIND-BODY-SPIRIT CONNECTION

Exploring how Grounding practices can facilitate a deeper connection between the mind, body, and spirit.

Modern science and traditional wisdom have converged on one point: the mind, body, and spirit are interconnected, forming a complex, dynamic system that shapes our health and well-being. Practices that can nurture this connection and promote harmony between these three aspects are increasingly recognized as integral to maintaining optimal wellness. Grounding, also known as earthing, is one such practice. By establishing a direct connection with the Earth, grounding can potentially help foster a deeper alignment between the mind, body, and spirit. This exploration delves into how grounding might facilitate this connection.

Understanding the Mind-Body-Spirit Connection

The concept of mind-body-spirit connection arises from an understanding that our mental, physical, and spiritual well-being are intricately linked. Our thoughts and emotions can impact our physical health, just as physical conditions can influence our mental state. Spirituality, whether expressed as a connection to a higher power, a sense of purpose, or a deep appreciation of life, also significantly contributes to overall well-being.

Integrative and holistic healing modalities emphasize this connection and seek to address imbalances in any of these aspects that may contribute to health issues. The ultimate aim is to attain harmony between the mind, body, and spirit, which can lead to a more balanced, healthy, and fulfilling life.

Grounding: A Bridge Between the Natural World and Ourselves

Grounding is a practice that involves making a physical connection with the Earth, usually by walking barefoot outdoors or through other means like using grounding equipment. The Earth's surface carries a negative electrical charge, and direct contact with it allows the body to absorb this natural energy.

Grounding advocates suggest that this practice can yield numerous benefits, including reduced inflammation, improved sleep, and increased calm. As our ancestors were continually in contact with the Earth, grounding is seen as a way to restore our connection with nature, bringing our bodies back to their natural, balanced state.

Facilitating the Mind-Body-Spirit Connection through Grounding

Grounding's potential to deepen the connection between the mind, body, and spirit can be seen through its various reported benefits.

Body: Physical contact with the Earth can lead to the transfer of electrons into the body, contributing to the neutralization of free radicals and potentially reducing inflammation—an underlying factor in many chronic diseases. This could also enhance wound healing, reduce pain, and improve cardiovascular health.

Mind: Grounding can also support mental well-being. Exposure to nature and the physical act of grounding can create a sense of calm and help alleviate stress, anxiety, and depression. These positive effects on mental health can enhance clarity of thought and contribute to better emotional regulation.

Spirit: Grounding practices can strengthen our spiritual connection by promoting a sense of oneness with nature and the universe. This practice encourages us to be present in the moment, fostering mindfulness and a deeper appreciation of our place in the natural world.

Nurturing the Mind-Body-Spirit Connection with Grounding

Incorporating grounding into a daily routine can help nurture the mind-body-spirit connection over time. This could be as simple as taking a barefoot walk in the park, gardening, or meditating outdoors while in contact with the ground. Grounding can also be integrated with other mind-body-spirit practices such as yoga, tai chi, or mindfulness meditation, creating a holistic practice that simultaneously engages all three aspects.

Beyond Grounding: A Holistic Approach

While grounding can offer numerous benefits, it's important to remember that it is just one aspect of a comprehensive approach to nurturing the mind-body-spirit connection. Regular physical activity, balanced nutrition, adequate sleep, mental health care, and practices such as meditation, prayer, or other forms of spiritual expression, all contribute to the health of the whole person.

The Road Ahead

Grounding offers a promising avenue to foster a deeper mind-body-spirit connection. However, while there's a growing body of research supporting the benefits of grounding, more extensive and rigorous studies would further clarify its role within a holistic wellness framework.

Conclusion

The practice of grounding provides a tangible way to experience the interconnectedness of the mind, body, and spirit. Through our direct connection with the Earth, we can potentially enhance our physical well-being, cultivate mental and emotional balance, and deepen our spiritual connection to the world around us. As we continue to explore and understand the power of the mind-body-spirit connection, grounding may serve as a vital practice, grounding us not only to the Earth beneath our feet but also to the profound interplay of our minds, bodies, and spirits.

34. GROUNDING AND THE POWER OF COMMUNITY

Discussing the Benefits of Practicing Grounding in a Community Setting and Fostering a Sense of Belonging

Human beings are inherently social creatures. The power of community has shaped civilizations, fostering a sense of belonging and creating shared values, traditions, and experiences. In the context of health and wellness, communal activities can have transformative effects on individuals' mental, emotional, and physical well-being. This is particularly true for grounding—a practice that connects us to the earth and each other in profound ways. This article delves into the benefits of practicing grounding in a community setting and the unique sense of belonging it can foster.

Grounding as a Communal Practice

While grounding can be an individual practice, performing it in a community setting can bring added dimensions of shared experience, mutual support, and collective energy. Like yoga or meditation groups, a grounding community can provide a structure for regular practice, encouragement, and shared learning.

Shared Experience: Practicing grounding as a group can amplify the benefits of the activity by introducing the element of shared experience. Members can learn from each other's experiences, discuss insights, and collectively enhance their understanding of the practice and its impacts.

Mutual Support: A grounding community provides a platform for mutual support. Practitioners can motivate each other, share tips and strategies, and collectively navigate challenges. The encouragement and moral support within a community can be crucial for beginners and can sustain the practice over the long term.

Collective Energy: There is something powerful about collective intention and energy. Engaging in grounding as a group can amplify individual energies and intensify the overall grounding experience. This shared energy can contribute to a more profound connection with the Earth and with each other.

Grounding and the Sense of Belonging

The communal practice of grounding can also foster a strong sense of belonging. This feeling of being part of a group can significantly impact one's mental and emotional health.

Belonging to a community with shared interests can reinforce individual identity and self-esteem. Being part of a grounding group can offer the assurance that others value and understand one's experiences and perspectives. It provides a safe space for expressing thoughts and emotions related to the grounding practice, leading to deeper connections among group members.

Moreover, a grounding community can foster social connection, which is a fundamental human need. Strong social connections are associated with improved mental health, increased feelings of happiness, and lower levels of stress and anxiety. Participating in a grounding community can contribute to these beneficial social connections.

Creating a Grounding Community

Creating a grounding community can start with a few like-minded individuals committed to practicing together regularly. It could be as simple as a weekly meet-up in a local park for a barefoot walk or meditation session. Regular discussions or sharing sessions can also be incorporated to share experiences, challenges, and insights. As the community grows, more structured activities like grounding retreats, workshops, or guest speaker sessions can be organized to enrich the group's experience.

Grounding in the Digital Age

In today's digital age, grounding communities are not limited by geographical boundaries. Online platforms can be used to connect individuals from across the globe, fostering a global grounding community. These virtual communities can organize live grounding sessions, webinars, discussion forums, and other interactive activities to engage members and share the grounding practice.

Conclusion

Grounding as a communal practice harnesses the power of community to enhance individual and collective wellness. By connecting us with the Earth and each other, grounding communities foster a unique sense of belonging that uplifts and supports each member. As we increasingly recognize the interconnectedness of our health with our environment and social context, grounding offers an accessible practice that can be shared, enjoyed, and enriched within the embrace of a community.

35. GROUNDING AND THE POWER OF NATURE IMMERSION

Grounding and the Power of Nature Immersion: Investigating the Transformative Effects of Immersing Oneself in Nature and Grounding Practices.

The concept of grounding, also known as earthing, takes on a deeper meaning when it is viewed in the context of nature immersion. Our relationship with the natural environment is not simply passive; we interact with nature in ways that can have profound effects on our well-being. In this discourse, we delve into the transformative effects of grounding oneself in nature and the practices that enable this life-enhancing connection.

Understanding Grounding and Nature Immersion

Grounding is a practice that involves making direct physical contact with the earth. The science of grounding is based on the idea that the earth's electromagnetic field has a stabilizing and healing effect on our bodies. This grounding effect can be experienced through activities such as walking barefoot in the grass, sitting on the beach, or even just touching a tree.

Nature immersion, on the other hand, refers to spending time in the natural environment in a way that encourages active engagement and promotes a sense of being part of nature. This can range from forest bathing, a practice originated in Japan known as **Shinrin-Yoku**, to simply spending time in a garden or a park.

The Interconnection Between Grounding and Nature Immersion

Grounding and nature immersion are interconnected practices. They both involve engaging with the natural environment in a meaningful and mindful way. However, grounding places emphasis on physical contact with the earth, while nature immersion focuses on spending quality time in nature, taking in the surroundings with all the senses.

Grounding practices can enhance the experience of nature immersion by making it more tactile and visceral. It allows the individual to feel more connected to the earth, providing a direct physical link to the environment around them. On the other hand, nature immersion can deepen the grounding practice by engaging not just the physical, but also the emotional and cognitive facets of the individual.

The Transformative Effects of Grounding and Nature Immersion

Immersion in nature and grounding practices have been found to offer numerous physical and psychological benefits.

Physical Benefits: The physical contact with the earth in grounding practices has been linked to several health benefits. These include reduced inflammation, improved sleep, and increased energy levels. Nature immersion also offers physical benefits such as improved cardiovascular health due to the calming effects of being in a natural environment.

Psychological Benefits: Both grounding and nature immersion have been found to have significant psychological benefits. They help reduce stress, improve mood, and enhance cognitive functioning. The act of grounding can create feelings of stability and connectedness, while nature immersion promotes a sense of peace and tranquility.

Spiritual Benefits: The practices of grounding and nature immersion can also facilitate a deep spiritual connection with the earth. This can foster a sense of oneness with nature, cultivating feelings of gratitude, awe, and reverence for the natural world.

Environmental Benefits: Grounding and nature immersion encourage a greater appreciation for nature, which can inspire actions toward environmental conservation. The practices enhance our awareness of the interconnectedness of all life, reinforcing the need for sustainable living.

Enhancing Grounding and Nature Immersion Practices

To maximize the transformative effects of grounding and nature immersion, it is important to practice mindfulness during these activities. This involves focusing your attention on the present moment and observing your surroundings with all your senses. Whether it is feeling the texture of the earth beneath your feet, listening to the sounds of nature, or observing the colors and movements in your surroundings, mindfulness amplifies the connection to nature.

Additionally, regular practice is key. The more frequently you engage in grounding and nature immersion, the more attuned you become to the subtle changes in your environment and in your own body.

Conclusion

Grounding and nature immersion, when practiced together, offer a powerful means of enhancing our health, well-being, and relationship with the natural world. These practices remind us of our inherent connection to the earth, leading to transformative experiences that nourish our body, calm our mind, and feed our spirit. In a world where we are often disconnected from our natural environment, grounding and nature immersion provide avenues for reconnection, revitalization, and restoration.

36. GROUNDING AND THE POWER OF FOREST BATHING

Exploring the Japanese practice of forest bathing and its connection to Grounding.

Grounding, or earthing, and forest bathing, known as Shinrin-yoku in Japan, are two powerful practices that encourage a deep, healing connection with nature. Both offer a sanctuary from the fast-paced world, helping individuals connect with their roots and find balance and peace in nature's cradle. This discussion explores the profound relationship between these two practices, elucidating their healing power and mutual interplay.

Understanding Grounding and Forest Bathing

Grounding is the practice of making direct physical contact with the Earth's surface, such as walking barefoot on grass or soil. The Earth's surface holds a natural negative charge, and through this contact, it's believed that the body can absorb negative electrons, which can neutralize harmful free radicals and bring about a variety of health benefits.

On the other hand, Shinrin-yoku, which translates to "forest bathing" or "taking in the forest atmosphere," is a practice that encourages individuals to immerse themselves in nature and absorb the atmosphere through all their senses. Introduced in Japan in the 1980s, it has since gained global recognition for its potential physical, emotional, and psychological benefits.

The Connection Between Grounding and Forest Bathing

The convergence of grounding and forest bathing is essentially a communion with nature. Grounding can be seen as the physical aspect of this communion, while forest bathing involves a deeper, sensory immersion in the forest atmosphere. The shared principle between the two is their basis on the healing power of nature, and they both foster a mindful connection with our natural surroundings.

When practicing forest bathing in a grounded state—such as walking barefoot on the forest floor or sitting against a tree—the forest's therapeutic elements are enhanced, fostering a more potent connection with the Earth. Through grounding during forest bathing, one can enjoy not only the sensory experience offered by the forest but also the health benefits associated with grounding.

The Healing Power of Grounding and Forest Bathing

Research into grounding has suggested potential benefits including reduced inflammation, improved sleep, decreased stress levels, and enhanced overall well-being. These results stem from the idea that grounding may balance the body's electrical energy, thus promoting health.

Similarly, forest bathing has been scientifically shown to strengthen the immune system, lower blood pressure, reduce stress, improve mood, increase energy levels, and improve sleep. Various elements contribute to these health benefits, including the visual calmness of nature, the smell of phytoncides (naturally occurring compounds emitted by plants), and the serene sounds of the forest.

When grounding is incorporated into forest bathing, these benefits may interact and enhance each other, facilitating a more comprehensive healing experience. This amalgamation offers a multi-sensory therapeutic approach—touching the earth, inhaling the forest's aroma, hearing the natural sounds, and seeing the verdant surroundings—that embraces the holistic concept of mind-body wellness.

Enhancing Grounding and Forest Bathing Practices

In both grounding and forest bathing, mindfulness plays a vital role in augmenting their potential benefits. Being present, aware, and engaged in the experience can heighten the sensory immersion and promote a more profound connection with nature. This involves consciously acknowledging the sensations against the skin, the sounds around, the sights, and the aromas of the forest, thus enabling a deeper appreciation of our natural environment.

Furthermore, consistency can also enhance the effects of grounding and forest bathing. Making these practices a regular part of one's lifestyle can contribute to long-term health benefits and a sustained sense of peace and balance.

Conclusion

The fusion of grounding and forest bathing provides a pathway for us to reconnect with nature on both a physical and sensory level. In today's rapidly advancing world, such practices offer a refuge, promoting physical health, mental tranquility, and spiritual grounding. As we move forward, nurturing our relationship with the Earth becomes not just an optional indulgence, but a necessary journey back to our roots, fostering balance, wellness, and harmony within and around us.

37. GROUNDING AND THE POWER OF WATER

Discussing the benefits of combining Grounding practices with water-based activities, such as swimming or hydrotherapy.

The concept of grounding, or earthing, and its connection to water may not be immediately apparent, but these two natural elements share a harmonious relationship that can be harnessed to enhance our health and well-being. Grounding is the practice of making direct contact with the Earth's surface to absorb its healing properties, while water-based activities like swimming and hydrotherapy offer their own therapeutic benefits. This exploration will delve into the intersection of these two practices, offering insights into their individual benefits and their potential synergies.

Grounding: A Nature-Based Therapeutic Practice

Grounding is a healing modality that harnesses the Earth's energy by encouraging direct contact with its surface. Walking barefoot on grass, lying on a sandy beach, or even just touching a tree can all be forms of grounding. It's based on the theory that the Earth possesses a natural charge, which we can tap into to neutralize harmful free radicals and restore balance in our body. Grounding is said to have numerous benefits, including reduced inflammation, improved sleep, and better overall mood.

Water-Based Activities: A Source of Physical and Mental Health

Water, in its myriad forms, offers a host of health and wellness benefits. Activities like swimming and hydrotherapy are renowned for their capacity to boost physical health, encourage relaxation, and promote emotional well-being. Swimming is a full-body workout, strengthening muscles, enhancing cardiovascular health, and improving flexibility. Moreover, the rhythmic nature of swimming strokes can have a calming, almost meditative effect.

Hydrotherapy, on the other hand, uses water's therapeutic properties for treatment purposes. The buoyancy, heat, and flow of water can help alleviate pain, improve circulation, encourage relaxation, and boost mood. Additionally, being in or around water has been linked to feelings of tranquility and happiness, a concept known as 'blue mind' in psychology.

Combining Grounding and Water-Based Activities

The relationship between grounding and water activities exists in the interplay of earth and water - two fundamental elements that hold unique healing properties. Whether it's walking barefoot along a beach, grounding while wading in a natural body of water, or practicing mindful connection to the Earth during a swim or hydrotherapy session, the intersection of grounding and water activities can be a potent source of physical and mental healing.

By grounding ourselves while we engage in water activities, we can tap into the Earth's energy even as we reap the benefits of the water. The negative ions present in natural bodies of water like oceans and lakes are believed to have a grounding effect similar to direct contact with the Earth. This allows us to double the health benefits - gaining the positive impacts of grounding and the therapeutic effects of water simultaneously.

The Synergy of Grounding and Water-Based Activities

Both grounding and water-based activities are known to alleviate stress, improve mood, and promote overall well-being. When combined, these benefits can synergize, potentially resulting in a more significant impact on mental and physical health.

In terms of physical benefits, grounding can boost recovery from the physical exertion of swimming, reducing inflammation and aiding muscle repair. Simultaneously, the strengthening and cardiovascular enhancements from swimming can complement grounding's health benefits.

Emotionally, the tranquility offered by both grounding and water activities can amplify feelings of peace, calm, and happiness. The 'blue mind' state associated with being near water can be heightened by grounding practices, offering deeper relaxation and a stronger connection to the natural world.

Furthermore, practicing mindfulness during these activities can augment their benefits. By consciously connecting with the sensations of water and the Earth, one can enhance their healing experience.

Conclusion

Grounding and water-based activities, when combined, present a holistic, natural approach to health and well-being. The synergistic relationship between these practices can create a potent form of therapy, capitalizing on the healing properties of both the Earth and water. In a world that often disconnects us from nature, these practices offer a pathway back to our roots, reminding us of the healing power that lies in our natural environment. Whether we are grounding on a sandy beach or immersing ourselves in the rhythmic cadence of swimming, these practices encourage us to embrace nature as our partner in health and wellness.

38. GROUNDING AND THE POWER OF SUNLIGHT

Investigating the relationship between Grounding and sunlight exposure for optimal health and vitality.

The integration of Grounding practices with sunlight exposure offers a remarkable synergy in promoting health and vitality. Grounding or earthing, which involves making a direct physical connection with the Earth, combined with the benefits of sunlight, can support both physical and emotional wellness. This exploration will delve into the benefits of each and highlight the potential for combining these two elements.

Grounding: The Earth's Healing Touch

Grounding refers to the simple yet powerful practice of physically connecting with the Earth, typically by going barefoot on natural surfaces like grass, sand, or soil. This practice is rooted in the understanding that the Earth emits a natural electromagnetic field, rich in free electrons, which we can absorb through our skin. Grounding is said to neutralize free radicals, reduce inflammation, enhance mood, and improve sleep quality, among other benefits. It is a holistic practice, aiming to restore our bodies to a more natural, balanced state.

The Power of Sunlight

Sunlight, meanwhile, holds its own array of health benefits. Exposure to sunlight triggers the skin's production of vitamin D, a vital nutrient that supports bone health, immune function, and mental well-being. In fact, deficiencies in **vitamin D** have been linked to various health issues, from depression to certain cancers.

Moreover, sunlight exposure has been shown to regulate our body's circadian rhythm, our internal "body clock" that governs sleep-wake cycles. Regular sunlight exposure, particularly in the morning, can help maintain a healthy sleep pattern and boost overall mood. In addition, sunlight has been reported to stimulate the production of serotonin, the "feel-good" hormone, potentially helping to ward off feelings of depression and anxiety.

Combining Grounding and Sunlight: A Pathway to Enhanced Health

When you merge the practice of Grounding with regular exposure to sunlight, a synergy occurs, creating a holistic approach to wellness. By grounding ourselves barefoot on the Earth while simultaneously soaking up sunlight, we can harness the Earth's energy and absorb the beneficial UVB rays from the sun, thereby doubling the health benefits.

Grounding and sunlight exposure both contribute to the reduction of inflammation, a key factor in many chronic diseases. The free electrons absorbed through Grounding can neutralize the excess free radicals that cause **oxidative stress** and inflammation in our bodies. Simultaneously, **vitamin D** produced through sunlight exposure has been shown to have **anti-inflammatory properties**.

Furthermore, both practices can enhance mood and mental well-being. Grounding can balance the autonomic nervous system, promoting relaxation and reducing stress, while sunlight can increase serotonin levels, contributing to feelings of happiness and calm.

Sleep regulation is another shared benefit. Grounding can help balance the circadian rhythm by aligning our bodies with the Earth's natural electromagnetic field, while morning sunlight exposure can reset our internal body clock, promoting regular sleep patterns and improving sleep quality.

An Integrated Approach to Health

Taking a comprehensive approach, combining Grounding with sunlight exposure, provides a well-rounded way to connect with our environment and tap into nature's healing mechanisms. These practices can be easily incorporated into our daily routines: morning walks barefoot on the grass while the sun is rising, or meditative sessions on a sandy beach in the gentle evening sunlight. These simple activities not only enhance our physical health but also offer an opportunity to foster a deeper connection with the Earth and the sun, grounding us in the present moment and promoting mental well-being.

The combination of Grounding and sunlight exposure offers a potent and accessible strategy for overall health and vitality. It's a reminder of the healing power of nature, and our inherent connection to the Earth and the sun. As we face increasing rates of lifestyle-related health conditions in our modern world, integrating these simple, natural practices into our daily routine may be one path towards enhanced health, vitality, and wellness. Ultimately, the combination of Grounding and sunlight exposure underscores the importance of our relationship with nature and the powerful impact this connection can have on our health and well-being.

39. GROUNDING AND THE POWER OF BREATH OF FRESH AIR

Exploring the benefits of fresh air and outdoor environments in conjunction with Grounding practices.

The benefits of fresh air and outdoor environments are widely recognized. Fresh air revitalizes us, invigorates our senses, and provides vital oxygen for our bodies. When these advantages are combined with grounding practices—wherein we directly connect with the Earth's surface—there's a potential for transformative wellness effects. This exploration sheds light on the dynamic interplay of grounding, fresh air, and outdoor settings, and their collective impact on our health and well-being.

The Benefits of Fresh Air

Fresh air plays a crucial role in our well-being, both physically and mentally. Physically, fresh air helps to cleanse the lungs, boost the immune system, and provide our bodies with a constant supply of oxygen, necessary for cell regeneration and vitality.

Mentally, stepping out into fresh air can clear the mind, reduce stress, and improve mood. Fresh air is often filled with negative ions, particularly around **areas like forests and bodies of water**, which are believed to produce biochemical reactions that increase **serotonin levels**, consequently uplifting mood and alleviating stress.

The Healing Power of Outdoor Environments

Beyond the physical and mental benefits, being in an outdoor environment has been linked with numerous positive health outcomes. Exposure to natural light, the visual stimulation of green spaces, the sounds of birdsong, or the rustling of leaves can all provide sensory benefits that contribute to our well-being. Research has even shown that **spending time in green spaces can lower heart rate, blood pressure, and levels of the stress hormone cortisol.**

Synergy of Grounding, Fresh Air, and the Outdoors

When we combine grounding with the benefits of fresh air and outdoor environments, we set the stage for a potent blend of health-promoting factors. Practicing grounding outdoors exposes us to fresh air, allowing us to simultaneously reap the rewards of both.

As we ground ourselves, the intake of fresh air enhances the experience and strengthens the benefits. The deep, mindful breathing often associated with grounding practices is a perfect match for the clean, oxygen-rich air found in outdoor settings, aiding in reducing stress levels and promoting a state of calm and relaxation.

Moreover, the outdoor environment serves to deepen the grounding experience. Visual stimuli from the surroundings, the feeling of the natural terrain under bare feet, and the auditory backdrop of nature, all contribute to a fuller, more immersive experience. This multisensory engagement not only enhances the grounding practice but also bolsters our overall connection with the natural world.

Incorporating Grounding and Fresh Air Into Your Routine

Incorporating grounding and fresh air into daily life doesn't require drastic changes. It could be as simple as taking a barefoot walk in the park during lunch, meditating in your garden in the early morning, or reading a book on the beach. The key is consistency and mindfulness—being present in the moment, consciously breathing in the fresh air, and physically connecting with the Earth.

In a world increasingly dominated by indoor living and screen time, grounding and taking in fresh air outdoors offers a counterbalance, bringing us back to our roots. This practice not only has potential health benefits but also allows us to forge a deeper connection with the natural world, fostering a greater appreciation for our environment.

In conclusion, the symbiotic relationship between grounding, fresh air, and outdoor environments presents a compelling case for an integrated approach to wellness—one that is accessible, natural, and deeply tied to our inherent connection with the Earth. The combination of these elements is a testament to the power of nature as a source of health, vitality, and well-being. As we navigate the challenges of the modern world, these simple yet profound practices may well serve as a foundation for holistic health and longevity.

40. GROUNDING AND THE POWER OF SACRED SPACES

Discussing the significance of creating sacred spaces for Grounding practices and spiritual connection.

The practice of grounding, or creating a physical connection with the Earth, has gained attention for its potential benefits to physical and emotional health. Equally important in the realm of holistic wellness is the concept of sacred spaces, areas that we designate as special and imbued with personal or spiritual significance. When grounding practices are performed within such spaces, there can be a profound amplification of the benefits experienced. This discussion delves into the importance of creating sacred spaces for grounding and explores their potential to enhance spiritual connectivity.

Understanding Grounding and Sacred Spaces

Sacred spaces, on the other hand, are areas set aside for spiritual reflection, meditation, or simply quiet contemplation. They can be places in nature, a dedicated corner of your home, or any place that holds spiritual significance for you. The creation of such spaces is deeply personal and can be as simple or complex as you wish, often involving elements that bring peace, inspire reflection, or carry personal or spiritual significance.

The Intersection of Grounding and Sacred Spaces

When grounding practices are integrated into sacred spaces, a powerful synergy can occur. The sacred space provides a calm and focused environment that enhances the grounding experience, while grounding within this space can strengthen the feeling of connection to the Earth and, by extension, the spiritual realm.

Grounding in a sacred space combines the physical and tangible experience of grounding with the more ethereal and personal aspect of spiritual connection. As you connect physically with the Earth through grounding, you may find a deeper spiritual connection with the universe and your higher self, amplified by the special significance of sacred space.

Creating a Sacred Space for Grounding

Creating a sacred space for grounding involves selecting a location and incorporating elements that have personal or spiritual significance. If possible, an outdoor space is ideal for grounding — perhaps a garden, a quiet corner of a yard, or even a balcony for those living in apartments. This space can be enhanced with elements such as plants, crystals, symbols, or anything that resonates with you on a personal level.

Importantly, a sacred space need not be large or extravagant. What matters is the intention behind the space and the sense of peace and connection it fosters. Once the space is created, it can serve as a dedicated place for grounding practices, meditation, or simply quiet reflection.

The Benefits of Grounding in a Sacred Space

Grounding in a sacred space can enhance both the grounding and the spiritual experience. As you connect physically with the Earth through grounding, the tranquil and personally significant environment of the sacred space can foster a deeper spiritual connection. Practice can become a ritual that grounds you not just physically, but also emotionally and spiritually.

Moreover, the routine of practicing grounding in the same sacred space can enhance the sense of ritual and significance, making the practice even more powerful over time. It provides a regular opportunity to disconnect from the demands of daily life and reconnect with the Earth and oneself in a meaningful and deliberate way.

In Conclusion: Grounding, Sacred Spaces, and Holistic Well-being

The interplay between grounding and sacred spaces underscores the holistic nature of well-being. Physical health does not exist in isolation; our emotional and spiritual health is intricately linked. By creating a sacred space for grounding, we acknowledge this interconnection and provide an avenue to nurture all aspects of our being.

Moreover, it also highlights the importance of intention in wellness practices. Creating a sacred space is an act of intention, signifying a commitment to personal well-being and spiritual growth. Similarly, grounding is not just about physical connection with the Earth, but also about being present and mindful.

Ultimately, the integration of grounding and sacred spaces offers a pathway to holistic wellness that is accessible to anyone, regardless of their spiritual beliefs or living situation. By honoring our need for physical connection with the Earth and our desire for spiritual connection, we can create a balanced and fulfilling approach to wellness.

41. GROUNDING AND THE POWER OF JOURNALING

Investigating how journaling can enhance the Grounding experience and promote self-reflection.

Grounding, or earthing, and journaling might seem to be disparate activities at first glance, but they intersect at a shared point - personal well-being. Grounding, involving direct physical contact with the earth's surface, encourages physical health by aiding in inflammation reduction, sleep improvement, and more. Journaling, on the other hand, promotes mental well-being by encouraging self-expression, mindfulness, and emotional release. By combining these two practices, individuals can experience an amplified sense of whole-person health and wellness. Let's dive into this unique synergy.

Understanding Grounding and Journaling

Journaling, on the other hand, is a reflective practice of recording thoughts, feelings, and experiences. It has been widely recognized for its mental health benefits, including reducing anxiety, aiding in stress management, and promoting mindfulness. Journaling can also foster personal growth and enhance self-awareness, as it allows one to process experiences and emotions in a tangible way.

The Interplay of Grounding and Journaling

When we combine grounding with journaling, the benefits of both practices can be amplified. Grounding serves as a physical connection to the Earth, enhancing our sense of being in the present moment and providing a tranquil environment for reflection. Meanwhile, journaling can translate these experiences into a tangible form, allowing us to understand and process our thoughts, feelings, and experiences more deeply.

The experience of grounding can offer rich material for journal entries. As one becomes more in tune with the physical sensations of grounding, such as the feel of the earth beneath one's feet, the sounds of nature, or the rhythm of one's breath, these can be explored and documented through journaling. This encourages mindfulness and presence, core aspects of both grounding and journaling.

Enhancing the Grounding Experience through Journaling

To integrate journaling into your grounding practice, consider bringing a notebook or journal with you when you ground. After spending some time grounding, sit quietly and write about your experience. Focus on your senses - what do you feel, hear, see, smell? How does your body feel? What emotions or thoughts emerged during your grounding practice?

Over time, this routine can enhance your grounding practice. Writing about your experiences helps you pay closer attention to them, cultivating a deeper sense of mindfulness. It can also provide valuable insights into your well-being and growth over time. You may notice patterns or changes that provide a deeper understanding of your connection with nature and your overall health.

The Benefits of Grounding and Journaling

The combination of grounding and journaling offers numerous benefits. Here are a few key advantages:

Enhanced Mindfulness: Both grounding and journaling promote mindfulness, or the practice of being fully present and engaged in the current moment. Combining these practices can enhance this effect, fostering a deeper connection with the self and the environment.

Emotional Release: Journaling provides an avenue for expressing and releasing emotions. When paired with the calming practice of grounding, it can be particularly effective in managing stress and anxiety.

Increased Self-awareness: As you record your grounding experiences and reflect on them, you can gain a better understanding of your emotional and physical states. This can lead to increased self-awareness and insights into personal growth and well-being.

Strengthened Connection with Nature: Writing about your grounding experiences can help you appreciate your connection with nature on a deeper level, fostering a greater sense of respect and care for the environment.

In conclusion, the combination of grounding and journaling provides a holistic approach to personal well-being, addressing both physical and mental health. As a grounding-journaling practitioner, you harness the Earth's natural energy while also exploring your inner thoughts and emotions, creating an overall sense of harmony and balance. This powerful practice can serve as a pathway to personal growth, mindfulness, and a deeper connection with the natural world.

42. GROUNDING AND THE POWER OF ART THERAPY

Exploring how artistic expression can be combined with Grounding practices for emotional healing and self-discovery.

Grounding, or Earthing, is a practice focused on reconnecting our bodies with the earth's natural energy to enhance physical and mental well-being. On the other hand, art therapy involves using creative mediums for therapeutic purposes, promoting mental health, and fostering self-discovery. When combined, grounding and art therapy can facilitate a deeply transformative process, enhancing both emotional healing and self-discovery. This unique blend creates a dynamic and potent practice with wide-ranging benefits. Let's delve into this fascinating confluence of Earth and Art.

The Interplay of Grounding and Art Therapy

Grounding and art therapy are both therapeutic practices that cater to different aspects of our well-being. Grounding focuses on physical well-being, harnessing the earth's natural energy to mitigate chronic inflammation, improve sleep, and reduce stress. It involves direct skin-to-earth contact, typically by walking barefoot on natural surfaces.

Art therapy, meanwhile, emphasizes mental and emotional health. It involves creating and reflecting on art, using the process as a means of self-expression, exploration, and healing. Art therapy can help individuals express feelings that they can't articulate, understand and resolve emotional conflicts, reduce anxiety, and improve self-esteem.

Bringing these two practices together creates an experience that nourishes both the body and mind. Grounding provides a physical and mental state conducive to artistic expression, and art therapy offers a means of expressing the mental and emotional shifts experienced during grounding.

Enhancing Grounding with Art Therapy

Combining grounding and art therapy can be as simple as taking art materials outdoors and creating while grounded. You can sit or stand barefoot on the ground while painting, drawing, sculpting, or engaging in any other art form. This allows you to harness the benefits of grounding as you engage in artistic creation, offering a sense of calmness and focus that can enhance creativity.

The outdoors itself can serve as an inspiration. The colors of the sky, the shape of the trees, the feel of the wind - these can all influence your art, leading to creations that truly capture your grounding experience. Additionally, using natural materials like leaves, rocks, or water from a stream can further enhance the connection between your art and the environment.

Benefits of Combining Grounding and Art Therapy

Combining grounding and art therapy results in several benefits that enhance emotional healing and self-discovery.

Increased Mindfulness: Both grounding and art therapy require presence and awareness, enhancing mindfulness and bringing you fully into the present moment. This can reduce stress, improve focus, and enhance overall well-being.

Improved Self-Expression: Art therapy offers a powerful means of self-expression. When grounded, you might find your art reflecting your emotional state more accurately, leading to greater understanding and acceptance of your feelings.

Emotional Healing: The combination of grounding and art therapy can promote emotional healing. Grounding reduces anxiety and stress, providing a calm state conducive to therapeutic art creation. Through art, you can process emotions, leading to improved mental health.

Enhanced Connection with Nature: Creating art while grounded can strengthen your connection with the environment, fostering a greater appreciation of nature's beauty and encouraging environmental stewardship.

Self-Discovery: Through the creative process, you can discover new aspects of your personality, preferences, and thoughts. This process of self-discovery can lead to personal growth and increased self-understanding.

Conclusion

Grounding and art therapy, when combined, offer a holistic approach to well-being. By engaging in artistic expression while grounded, you're not only nurturing your physical health through the earth's natural energy, but you're also promoting mental and emotional healing through the creative process. This practice brings together the healing energies of the Earth and the therapeutic power of art, creating a space for deep emotional healing and self-discovery. Thus, grounding and art therapy stand as testament to the fact that the pursuit of well-being can be as creative and unique as we allow it to be.

43. GROUNDING AND THE POWER OF DANCE

Discussing the benefits of incorporating Grounding practices into Power of Dance

The intersection of Grounding, or Earthing, and dance represents a unique symbiosis of physical movement and earthly connection that invites an exploration of self-expression, mindfulness, and holistic well-being. Grounding involves direct contact with the Earth's surface, inviting the absorption of its negative electrons into the body to balance the positive ions and promote a sense of wellness. Dance, a rhythmic manifestation of music and motion, is an artistic language that resonates deeply within the human spirit, serving as a medium of expression and a source of physical activity. When these two practices intertwine, they form a potent combination that harmonizes the mind, body, and spirit with the rhythms of the Earth.

A Dance on Earth: Blending Grounding and Dance

The integration of grounding practices into dance can be achieved in various ways. The first and simplest approach is through barefoot dancing on natural surfaces such as grass, sand, or soil. When the skin comes into direct contact with these surfaces, the grounding effect occurs, providing a unique sensory experience that goes beyond the conventional dancing environment.

The incorporation of nature-inspired movements and rhythms can also augment the grounding effect. This can involve imitating the swaying of trees, the ebb and flow of the ocean, or the soaring of birds. Such movements deepen the connection with the natural world and foster a sense of being an integral part of it.

Outdoor dance performances or classes are other ways to facilitate this interaction between grounding and dance. Dancing in open-air environments not only provides ample opportunities for grounding but also allows dancers to feel the elements – the warmth of the sun, the breeze of the wind, the solidity of the earth – enhancing the overall experience.

Health and Wellness in Motion: The Benefits of Grounding and Dance

The marriage of grounding and dance brings forth an array of mental, physical, and emotional benefits.

Boosted Physical Health: The combination of grounding and dance contributes to improved physical health. Grounding has been associated with reduced inflammation, improved sleep, and enhanced wound healing. Meanwhile, dance, as a form of physical exercise, increases cardiovascular fitness, strengthens muscles, improves balance and coordination, and promotes overall body health.

Emotional Wellness: Dancing is often considered a cathartic experience, allowing for the expression of emotions that might be difficult to articulate otherwise. Coupled with grounding, which can help reduce stress and anxiety, the practice provides a potent therapy for emotional wellness.

Mind-Body Connection: Dance inherently demands a strong connection between the mind and body, requiring focus, coordination, and rhythm. Grounding deepens this connection, fostering a heightened sense of body awareness, a state of mindfulness, and a deeper understanding of one's physical presence in the world.

Enhanced Creativity: The synergistic action of grounding and dance can stimulate creativity. The sensory input from grounding, the emotional release from dance, and the mindful state created by both practices can act as catalysts for innovative movement, choreography, and self-expression.

Social Connection: Participating in dance classes or performances can promote social interaction, communication, and a sense of community. The shared experience of grounding and dancing together can foster deeper connections among participants, nurturing a supportive and inclusive environment.

Final Thoughts: The Dance of Life and Earth

Incorporating grounding into dance rituals brings a new dimension to the art of movement. It is not only about connecting with the Earth physically but also about embracing its rhythm, embodying its essence, and expressing it through the dance. The powerful combination of grounding and dance offers a holistic approach to wellness, providing physical health benefits, emotional release, and enhanced creativity. It encourages an intimate dance with nature, one where we listen to the Earth's rhythms and echo them with our bodies. In the dance of life, grounding provides the stage – the earth beneath our feet – making each movement a step towards greater health, harmony, and self-expression.

44. GROUNDING AND ADDICTION RECOVERY

Exploring the Potential Benefits of Grounding Practices for Individuals in Addiction Recovery.

Redo intro-In the complex and challenging journey of addiction recovery, grounding techniques can play a transformative role. Grounding, also known as Earthing, involves direct contact with the Earth's surface, allowing the body to absorb its naturally occurring negative ions, which can have significant health benefits. When applied to addiction recovery, grounding may serve as a crucial tool for those seeking to regain control over their lives and achieve sustained sobriety.

Understanding Addiction and Recovery

Addiction is a chronic brain disorder characterized by compulsive drug seeking and use, despite harmful consequences. It disrupts the reward system in the brain, making it difficult for individuals to stop using substances or engaging in certain behaviors. Recovery is a multifaceted process that requires physical healing, mental restoration, and emotional resilience. It demands a holistic approach that encompasses lifestyle changes, psychological support, medical intervention, and the cultivation of coping mechanisms.

Introducing Grounding in the Recovery Process

Incorporating grounding practices into the recovery process is an integrative approach that supports the body's natural healing capabilities. The grounding process, whether achieved through walking barefoot on the earth, grounding mats, or other grounding equipment, allows the body to tap into the Earth's energy, which can help balance the body's internal electrical environment and promote physical well-being.

Grounding and Physical Health in Recovery

The physical health benefits of grounding can be particularly advantageous during the detoxification phase of recovery. Grounding has been associated with reduced inflammation, improved sleep, increased energy levels, and better immune response, all of which are crucial in aiding the body's recovery from substance abuse. By helping to alleviate physical withdrawal symptoms and strengthening the body's ability to heal itself, grounding can contribute to a smoother and more manageable detox process.

Grounding and Emotional Regulation

Besides physical health, grounding can also be a powerful tool for emotional regulation. Addiction is often accompanied by heightened stress levels and emotional instability. Grounding can induce a state of calm, reduce stress, and promote a balanced mood by moderating cortisol, the body's primary stress hormone. Grounding can help individuals in recovery manage anxiety and depression symptoms, thus reducing the risk of relapse linked to emotional distress.

Grounding and Mindfulness

Grounding practices can enhance mindfulness - the ability to be present and fully engaged with the current moment. Developing mindfulness skills through grounding can help individuals in recovery break the cycle of automatic reactions that often leads to substance use. By fostering a greater awareness of thoughts, emotions, and physical sensations, grounding can empower individuals to respond to cravings or triggers in a more controlled and considered manner.

Grounding and Connection

Addiction can lead to feelings of isolation and disconnection from the self, others, and the environment. Grounding provides a physical connection to the Earth, which can foster a sense of belonging and re-establish a person's bond with nature. This connection can also serve as a metaphor for reconnection to one's body and the larger community, both of which are integral elements of recovery.

Final Thoughts: Grounding as a Recovery Tool

Incorporating grounding practices into the process of addiction recovery holds potential for enhancing the physical, emotional, and psychological aspects of healing. While grounding is not a standalone solution for addiction, it can be a powerful complementary tool in a comprehensive treatment plan. It serves to remind individuals in recovery of their innate connection to the world and their inherent potential for healing and transformation.

As with any integrative therapy, it's important for individuals in recovery to seek professional guidance and discuss the potential benefits and applicability of grounding practices in their specific recovery journey. Addiction recovery is a highly individualized process, and what works best will vary from person to person. However, grounding, as a natural and accessible practice, is a resource worth exploring in the path towards recovery and wellness.

45. GROUNDING ANDTRAUMA HEALING

Discussing How Grounding Practices Can Support Trauma Healing and Emotional Regulation

The healing journey from trauma can be a challenging and complex process. It involves addressing not only the psychological effects of traumatic experiences but also the physical and emotional responses. Among the myriad therapeutic approaches available, grounding practices hold promise as a potent, holistic, and self-empowering tool for trauma recovery and emotional regulation.

Understanding Trauma and its Impact

Trauma occurs when an individual experiences an event or series of events that they perceive as physically or emotionally harmful or life-threatening. It can leave a lasting impact on the person's mental, physical, and emotional health, often leading to post-traumatic stress disorder (PTSD), anxiety, depression, and other related conditions. Trauma disrupts the body's natural equilibrium, prompting the need for practices that can restore balance and promote healing.

Grounding and Physical Health in Trauma Healing

Physical health and trauma are inextricably linked. Trauma can manifest physically as chronic pain, inflammation, or tension. Research has suggested that grounding can help reduce inflammation and improve sleep, contributing to the body's overall healing process. By harmonizing the body's natural electrical state, grounding can alleviate physical symptoms and boost the body's healing capabilities.

Grounding and Emotional Regulation

A significant part of trauma healing involves managing and regulating intense emotional responses. Grounding practices can have a stabilizing effect on the body's bioelectrical environment, which in turn can influence emotional regulation. The direct connection with the Earth can induce a sense of calm and reduce stress levels by moderating the production of cortisol, the body's primary stress hormone. This practice can be particularly beneficial for individuals with trauma, aiding in the management of anxiety and depression symptoms.

Grounding and Mind-Body Connection

Grounding promotes a deepened mind-body connection, an essential aspect of trauma healing. Trauma often leads to disconnection or dissociation, where a person feels detached from their body or reality. Grounding exercises can help individuals regain a sense of presence and awareness, facilitating reconnection to their physical being. This practice enables individuals to be more attuned to their physical sensations, grounding them in the present moment and aiding in the release of traumatic energy stored in the body.

Grounding and Resilience

Resilience, the ability to adapt and bounce back from adversity, is a key factor in trauma recovery. Grounding, by virtue of its stress-reducing and mood-stabilizing effects, can support resilience-building. It offers a readily accessible tool for individuals to manage stressors and triggers in their environment, fostering a sense of control and self-efficacy that is critical for resilience.

Final Thoughts: Grounding as a Trauma Recovery Tool

While grounding is not a standalone cure for trauma, it can be a powerful adjunctive practice within a comprehensive treatment plan. Its potential benefits for physical health, emotional regulation, mind-body connection, and resilience can make it a valuable tool for individuals navigating the challenging path of trauma recovery.

As always, it is important to consult with healthcare professionals or therapists when integrating new practices like grounding into a trauma recovery regimen. Grounding can provide a natural, accessible resource in the trauma healing process, complementing traditional therapy and medication, and contributing to a holistic approach to recovery and well-being. Grounding practices remind us of our innate capacity for healing and our essential connection to the natural world, supporting the journey towards resilience and emotional health.

46. GROUNDING AND THE POWER OF MIND-BODY CONNECTION

Investigating How Grounding Practices Can Facilitate a Deeper Mind-Body Connection and Promote Overall Well-Being

The mind-body connection is an intrinsic part of human life. This link suggests that our emotions, thoughts, and attitudes can positively or negatively affect our biological functioning. Conversely, what we do with our physical bodies (what we eat, how much we exercise, even our posture) can impact our mental state. Among the various techniques to enhance this vital connection, Grounding, also known as Earthing, plays a noteworthy role.

Understanding the Mind-Body Connection

The idea of the mind-body connection refers to the intimate relationship between our mental and physical health. Modern science now supports what ancient healing traditions have known for centuries - that the mind and body are intricately connected, with our thoughts, feelings, beliefs, and attitudes having a direct effect on our physical health, and vice versa.

This understanding challenges the traditional biomedical model of health that views the mind and body as separate entities. Instead, it promotes a holistic view of health, where physical health cannot be separated from mental health. Any disruption in one invariably affects the other.

Grounding and the Physical Body

Grounding practices have been shown to deliver a range of physical health benefits. These include reducing inflammation, improving sleep, increasing energy, lowering stress, and enhancing circulation. The underlying theory suggests that direct contact with the Earth enables people to absorb free electrons, which neutralize harmful free radicals and reduce the oxidative stress associated with disease development.

Grounding and the Mind

Beyond its physical benefits, Grounding can also have profound effects on our mental health. The grounding effect is believed to influence the autonomic nervous system, leading to relaxation, improved mood, and decreased stress. By promoting a calm state of mind, Grounding allows for decreased nervous system arousal and provides an environment conducive to lower stress hormone levels.

Bridging the Gap: Grounding and Mind-Body Connection

Grounding serves as a bridge between our physical bodies and our mental state, promoting an enhanced mind-body connection. Grounding reminds us that we are not disconnected entities floating through life separately from the world around us. Instead, it allows us to feel more anchored and in touch with our physical bodies.

By doing so, Grounding can assist us in being more present in the moment, allowing for enhanced awareness and mindfulness. This is particularly beneficial for those dealing with issues such as anxiety or chronic stress, where disconnection from the present moment can contribute to their symptoms.

Moreover, the practice of Grounding encourages individuals to spend time in nature, promoting mindfulness, decreasing stress levels, and reducing symptoms of many mental health disorders. This time in nature serves as a reminder of our place in the larger ecosystem of life and can provide a sense of perspective that is therapeutic in and of itself.

Final Thoughts: Grounding for Holistic Well-being

In conclusion, Grounding represents a powerful practice for promoting a deeper mind-body connection. This connection is a cornerstone of overall well-being and resilience. It's a reminder that our bodies are not just vehicles for our brains but are intricately tied to our thoughts, feelings, and perceptions of the world around us.

By consciously fostering this connection through Grounding, we can promote both our physical and mental health. Regular grounding practices can not only provide significant benefits to our physical health but also encourage a state of mindfulness and presence that is essential for mental well-being.

Grounding can be easily incorporated into our daily routines - it requires no special equipment (though grounding products can enhance the experience) and can be as simple as taking a barefoot walk in the grass. This simple act can serve as a catalyst for improved health, greater mindfulness, and a deeper connection to the natural world. As such, it's a powerful tool for enhancing the essential mind-body connection and promoting holistic well-being.

47. GROUNDING AND THE POWER OF INTENTION

Exploring How Intention-Setting Can Enhance the Grounding Experience and Promote Manifestation

The practice of Grounding, or Earthing, is a potent tool for enhancing well-being, improving health, and promoting a deep connection with the Earth's energy. However, when combined with the power of intention, Grounding can transcend the physical realm and help manifest our desires into reality. This fusion of intention-setting and Grounding can lead to profound transformations in our lives, bringing us closer to our true selves and aligning us with our life's purpose.

When you ground yourself — by walking barefoot, hugging a tree, or using Grounding tools — you tap into the Earth's natural, restorative energy. This energy interaction is believed to promote physiological changes that contribute to overall wellness, including reduction in inflammation, pain, and stress, improved sleep, increased energy, and improved circulation.

Understanding the Power of Intention

Intention-setting is a powerful technique that involves projecting your thoughts, desires, and goals into the universe with the expectation that they will manifest in your life. The theory behind intention-setting is that our thoughts create our reality, and by aligning our thoughts with our desires, we can manifest what we truly want in our lives.

This approach is rooted in the law of attraction, which proposes that like attracts like. Positive thoughts attract positive outcomes, and negative thoughts yield undesirable results. Therefore, setting clear and positive intentions is seen as a way to consciously steer our lives in the direction we want them to go.

Grounding and Intention-Setting: The Intersection

Grounding and intention-setting can seamlessly blend into a powerful practice. When we ground ourselves, we align with the Earth's energy, stabilizing our own energy and creating a firm foundation. From this place of stability and alignment, setting intentions can become a much more potent practice.

During Grounding, our bodies become conductors of Earth's energy, allowing us to tap into the inherent rhythms of nature. This deep connection can create a state of mindfulness and presence, providing an ideal environment for setting intentions.

When we're grounded, our minds are more attuned to our thoughts, emotions, and desires. From this clear, focused state, we can set intentions that are genuinely aligned with our deepest desires and life's purpose. The grounded mind, unclouded by the noise of everyday life, can then project these intentions into the universe with more force and clarity.

Enhancing Grounding Experience with Intention

While Grounding in itself can provide significant physical and mental benefits, incorporating intention-setting can elevate the Grounding experience. Before starting a Grounding session, take a few moments to clear your mind and focus on your intention. It can be a simple phrase or a clear picture of what you want to manifest in your life.

As you ground yourself, visualize the Earth's energy as a supportive force that amplifies your intentions. Imagine this energy merging with your intention, giving it the strength and power to manifest in your life.

Post Grounding, make a habit of revisiting your intentions throughout the day, re-energizing them with your thoughts and emotions. The more energy you give to your intentions, the more likely they are to manifest in your life.

The Power of Manifestation

The act of manifestation is much more than wishful thinking. It's a process of bringing your thoughts, ideas, and goals into physical reality through your actions, beliefs, and attitudes. When Grounding is combined with setting intentions, the power to manifest is heightened. Grounding, in its essence, allows us to tap into the Earth's abundant energy source, which can serve to magnify our intentions and accelerate their manifestation.

In Conclusion

Grounding, coupled with the power of intention, can serve as a robust framework for personal transformation. By harnessing the Earth's energy and channeling our deepest desires and goals, we can create a tangible path towards achieving them. Whether your intentions are related to health, relationships, career, or personal growth, integrating Grounding and intention-setting can guide your journey and help bring your desires to fruition. Through this practice, we not only reap the physical benefits of Grounding but also empower ourselves to consciously shape our lives.

48. GROUNDING AND THE POWER OF AFFECTION

Discussing the Benefits of Physical Touch and Affection in Conjunction with Grounding Practices

The art of Grounding, also known as Earthing, reconnects us to the Earth's vital energy through direct contact with its surface. When this natural, restorative practice is combined with the power of affection and physical touch, we can enhance our well-being, foster deeper connections, and create more balanced lives. This amalgamation of Grounding and affection extends beyond just the physical benefits and delves into the emotional and psychological well-being of individuals.

Understanding the Concept of Grounding

Grounding is a holistic practice that encourages a direct connection with the Earth's surface. Whether you're walking barefoot on the grass, sitting against a tree, or employing a Grounding device, the objective is to tap into the Earth's inherent negative charge. This process is believed to counteract the positive charges accumulated in our bodies due to modern living and environmental factors, leading to a balanced internal bioelectrical environment.

Grounding has been associated with numerous health benefits, such as reduced inflammation, improved sleep, decreased stress, enhanced immunity, and increased energy. However, when we introduce the power of affection into this equation, we can amplify these benefits and foster deeper human connections.

The Power of Affection

Affection, particularly in the form of physical touch, is a fundamental human need. It plays a crucial role in our physical and emotional health, strengthening relationships, providing comfort, and reducing stress. Physical touch triggers the release of oxytocin, often referred to as the 'bonding hormone' or 'love hormone'. This hormone contributes to feelings of trust, bonding, and empathy, strengthening interpersonal relationships.

Physical touch also activates the vagus nerve, which plays a significant role in our body's rest-and-digest response, lowering heart rate and blood pressure and reducing stress and anxiety. Studies have also shown that physical touch, such as hugging or handholding, can reduce pain and boost the immune system.

Grounding and Affection: A Powerful Combination

Combining Grounding with affectionate physical touch can lead to a synergy of benefits. Grounding naturally calms the nervous system and reduces inflammation in the body, creating an ideal physiological state to receive the benefits of affection.

When we ground ourselves and engage in affectionate touch, we're leveraging two potent natural forces. Imagine sharing a grounding session with a loved one, where you're both barefoot on the earth, holding hands, or hugging. The physical contact with the Earth and with each other can heighten the shared experience, intensifying the feelings of connection, love, and empathy.

Moreover, shared Grounding sessions can become a sacred space for expressing affection and fostering deeper relationships. This practice can promote open communication, mutual understanding, and an enhanced sense of belonging. It's an opportunity to not only connect with the Earth but also to nurture our connections with each other, contributing to a balanced and harmonious life.

Enhancing Grounding with Affection

The concept of combining Grounding and affection revolves around the idea that, as social creatures, our relationships and connections with others are just as important as our connection with the Earth. To enhance your Grounding experience with affection, consider incorporating elements of physical touch into your practice. This can be as simple as holding hands with a loved one while walking barefoot in the park or hugging a friend or partner during a shared Grounding session.

The added layer of physical touch brings an element of warmth, trust, and togetherness to the Grounding experience. It creates a shared experience that not only enhances our connection to the Earth but also to each other.

Implications for Mental and Emotional Well-being

While Grounding has distinct physical benefits, the addition of affectionate touch introduces a profound impact on mental and emotional well-being. Affection can alleviate feelings of isolation, loneliness, and stress, promote feelings of safety and trust, and contribute to overall happiness. When combined with Grounding, these benefits are amplified, fostering a holistic sense of well-being that encompasses the physical, emotional, and relational aspects of our lives.

In Conclusion

The power of Grounding and affection underscores the interconnectedness of all aspects of our well-being – physical, emotional, relational, and environmental. By incorporating affectionate touch into our Grounding practices, we not only enhance our connection to the Earth's healing energy but also to each other, promoting a sense of wholeness, harmony, and love. The amalgamation of Grounding and the power of affection demonstrates that our health and happiness are intrinsically linked to our relationships with the Earth and with each other.

49. GROUNDING AND THE POWER OF SELF-CARE

Investigating How Grounding Practices Can Be Incorporated into Self-Care Routines for Enhanced Well-being

The practice of grounding, also known as earthing, involves making direct contact with the Earth's surface. This natural, restorative practice combined with self-care is a potent duo that fosters mental, emotional, and physical well-being. By integrating grounding into our self-care routines, we harness the Earth's healing energy and use it to fuel our pursuit of balanced health and peace of mind.

Grounding: A Natural Path to Well-being

Grounding taps into the Earth's inherent negative charge. It's believed that this negative charge can counteract the positive charges that our bodies accumulate due to environmental factors and modern living. When our feet touch the ground, we invite a natural exchange of energy between our bodies and the Earth, which can create a balanced internal bioelectrical environment.

Research indicates that grounding may have numerous health benefits. These include reduced inflammation, improved sleep quality, decreased stress, enhanced immunity, and an increased sense of overall well-being. Grounding offers a way to return to our roots and reconnect with nature, reminding us that we are a part of a larger ecosystem.

Self-Care: Essential for Health and Happiness

Self-care is the practice of taking action to preserve or improve one's health. It's about recognizing our needs and taking the time to meet them. Self-care can manifest in various ways, such as maintaining a healthy diet, exercising regularly, engaging in mindfulness or relaxation techniques, spending time with loved ones, pursuing hobbies, and ensuring we get enough rest.

While self-care is often associated with physical health, it's equally critical for our mental and emotional health. By taking care of our bodies, minds, and spirits, we can better cope with stress, enhance our self-esteem, and foster resilience. In essence, self-care is a vital strategy for maintaining balance and promoting overall well-being.

Grounding and Self-Care: A Harmonious Union

Integrating grounding into our self-care routines provides a unique opportunity to reconnect with our natural environment and ourselves. The act of grounding can be seen as a form of self-care in itself, fostering a sense of calm, balance, and connection that extends beyond the physical to the mental and emotional realms.

Here are some ways to integrate grounding into your self-care routine:

Barefoot Walks: One of the simplest ways to practice grounding is by walking barefoot on the Earth, whether it's on grass, sand, or soil. This activity can be a mindful and therapeutic experience, inviting you to feel the textures beneath your feet, breathe in fresh air, and absorb the surrounding natural beauty.

Outdoor Meditation: Incorporating grounding into your meditation routine can amplify the experience. Sit or lie on the ground while meditating, allowing your body to absorb the Earth's energy as your mind finds peace and clarity.

Grounding Exercises: Specific grounding exercises, such as visualizing roots extending from your feet into the Earth, can help anchor your energy and promote a sense of stability and calm.

Nature Immersion: Spend time in natural settings as part of your self-care routine, whether it's reading a book by a tree, gardening, or simply enjoying a picnic on the grass.

Sleep: Use grounding sheets or mats while sleeping to facilitate a continuous connection with the Earth's energy, potentially improving sleep quality and reducing inflammation and pain.

The Benefits of Grounding as Self-Care

The combination of grounding and self-care can lead to a heightened sense of well-being. Grounding can boost the physical benefits of self-care routines by improving sleep quality, reducing pain, and boosting immunity. In turn, this can have positive effects on mental and emotional health, such as reducing stress, enhancing mood, and fostering a deeper sense of connection with oneself and the natural world.

By incorporating grounding into self-care routines, we create opportunities for mindfulness and relaxation. Grounding can become a time for introspection and self-reflection, providing a space where we can connect with our inner selves, listen to our bodies, and acknowledge our feelings and emotions.

In Conclusion

The integration of grounding and self-care underscores the significance of holistic wellness approaches. It acknowledges the importance of our connection to the Earth and the profound effects this can have on our health and well-being. Through grounding, we can strengthen our self-care routines, cultivating a sense of peace and balance that resonates within our bodies, minds, and spirits. This harmonious blend of self-care and grounding serves as a reminder that our well-being is deeply rooted in our connection to the Earth and ourselves.

50. GROUNDING AND THE POWER OF SELF-COMPASSION

Discussing How Grounding Practices Can Support Self-Compassion and Self-Love

Grounding, an elemental practice that involves making direct contact with the earth's surface, offers a deep and enriching path to self-compassion and self-love. This powerful combination of grounding and self-compassion promotes holistic wellness and fosters a stronger sense of self-awareness, love, and acceptance.

Grounding: An Intrinsic Connection to Earth

The practice of grounding is believed to have profound effects on physical, mental, and emotional well-being. By connecting with the earth, either barefoot or through a conductive material, we expose ourselves to the earth's natural electrical field. This connection facilitates a transfer of negatively charged electrons from the earth to our bodies, which is said to neutralize positively charged free radicals associated with inflammation and disease.

Research suggests that grounding can improve sleep, reduce inflammation, promote relaxation, and boost overall well-being. It reconnects us to nature, reminding us that we are an integral part of the earth's ecosystems and a participant in the grand cycle of life.

Self-Compassion: A Vital Element of Personal Well-being

Self-compassion involves treating ourselves with kindness and understanding, especially during moments of failure or suffering.

It's a conscious effort to avoid harsh self-judgment and to instead embrace our vulnerabilities with warmth and acceptance.

Research has shown that self-compassion can contribute to increased resilience, lower levels of anxiety and depression, and improved emotional well-being. It encourages us to view our struggles as part of the universal human experience, rather than as an isolated event.

Grounding and Self-Compassion: A Harmonious Duo

The integration of grounding and self-compassion can produce a profound sense of peace and self-acceptance. The process of grounding itself can be seen as an act of self-compassion, a commitment to our well-being.

Grounding allows us to forge a stronger connection to our physical bodies. It offers an opportunity to tune into our physical sensations, acknowledge our emotional state, and be present in the moment. This mindfulness aspect of grounding aligns perfectly with self-compassion, which calls for heightened self-awareness and acknowledgment of our feelings without judgment.

Integrating Grounding into a Self-Compassion Practice

Grounding Meditation: Incorporate grounding into your meditation sessions by sitting or lying on the earth's surface. Envision the earth's energy entering your body, calming your mind, and soothing your emotions.

Mindful Walks: Walking barefoot on grass, sand, or soil can be a grounding and mindful practice. Feel the textures beneath your feet and observe your environment with a sense of awe and appreciation.

Nature Immersion: Spend time in nature as a form of grounding. Whether it's sitting under a tree, gardening, or hiking, these activities allow you to be present and in tune with the earth and yourself.

Grounding Yoga: Practice yoga outdoors on the earth's surface to combine the grounding benefits of earth connection with the self-awareness and self-compassion fostered through yoga.

Journaling: After a grounding session, journal about your experiences and emotions. This can provide a deeper insight into your feelings and promote a heightened sense of self-compassion.

The Ripple Effects of Grounding and Self-Compassion

Grounding and self-compassion, when practiced together, can lead to enhanced physical, mental, and emotional well-being. Grounding can enhance the physical benefits of self-compassion by improving sleep quality, reducing stress, and boosting immunity. Meanwhile, self-compassion encourages us to approach the grounding practice with a loving and accepting mindset, enriching the experience and our relationship with ourselves.

Grounding offers a sense of calm and tranquility that can aid in cultivating self-compassion. It allows us to be present and aware, providing a non-judgmental space to acknowledge our feelings and extend kindness towards ourselves.

Conclusion

The synergy between grounding and self-compassion underscores the multifaceted nature of holistic wellness. Grounding serves as a reminder that our well-being is deeply rooted in our connection with the earth and ourselves. Meanwhile, self-compassion teaches us to meet ourselves with kindness and understanding, especially during moments of struggle or discomfort.

Together, grounding and self-compassion foster a sense of deep self-awareness and acceptance, encouraging us to love ourselves more fully and genuinely. This harmonious blend of practices provides a robust foundation for personal growth and well-being, reminding us of our innate capacity for self-love and the healing power of our connection with the earth.

51. GROUNDING AND THE POWER OF FORGIVENESS

Exploring how Grounding Practices Can Support the Process of Forgiveness and Emotional Healing

Grounding, the practice of physically connecting with the earth to draw upon its natural energy, and forgiveness, the process of letting go of resentment and anger towards oneself or others, might seem like disparate concepts at first glance. However, when explored more deeply, these practices intersect in unique and profound ways, providing a synergistic pathway to emotional healing and personal growth.

Grounding: A Connection with Earth's Natural Energy

Grounding is based on the premise that our bodies are meant to be in contact with the earth, thereby drawing from its natural healing energy. This contact, whether it's walking barefoot on the grass or swimming in a natural body of water, allows us to tap into the earth's electrical charge, which is believed to neutralize free radicals in our bodies, reduce inflammation, and promote overall wellness.

Grounding provides a calming, balancing effect on our physical and emotional state. It encourages us to be present in the moment, grounding our thoughts and emotions in the physical sensations we experience. This awareness can be beneficial in the process of forgiveness, as it promotes mindfulness and emotional clarity.

Forgiveness: A Pathway to Emotional Healing

Forgiveness is a personal journey that involves letting go of resentment, anger, and hurt towards oneself or others. It doesn't mean forgetting the harm caused or excusing the offense, but rather choosing to free oneself from the burden of these negative emotions.

Research shows that forgiveness can lead to improved mental health, better relationships, and increased life satisfaction. It can lower stress, reduce symptoms of depression, and enhance our ability to connect with others. However, forgiveness can often be a difficult process that requires self-reflection, patience, and, above all, self-compassion.

Intersection of Grounding and Forgiveness

Grounding can provide a supportive environment for the process of forgiveness to unfold. It can help anchor us in the present moment and open up a space for introspection and emotional processing. The physical connection to the earth can serve as a potent metaphor for the release of negative emotions, symbolizing the process of letting go.

Grounding techniques can offer a way to manage the overwhelming emotions that might arise during the process of forgiveness. By focusing on the physical sensations of grounding, such as the feeling of the earth under our feet, we can create a safe distance from our emotional pain, providing a calm and neutral space to process our feelings.

Grounding Techniques for Forgiveness

Grounding Meditation: Meditating in a grounded state, perhaps sitting, or lying down outside, can create a calming environment for introspection. Envision the earth's energy entering your body and the release of negative emotions back into the earth.

Mindful Walks: Engage in grounding walks, paying attention to the sensation of each foot touching the ground. With each step, imagine releasing a bit of your resentment or pain.

Grounding Visualization: Use visualization to enhance your grounding practice. Imagine roots growing from your feet into the earth, drawing up nourishing energy, and releasing the burden of negative emotions.

Nature Connection: Spending time in nature can be grounding and restorative. Embrace the tranquility of nature and use this peaceful environment to reflect on your feelings and work towards forgiveness.

The Ripple Effect of Grounding and Forgiveness

The combination of grounding and forgiveness can lead to a state of enhanced emotional well-being. Grounding provides a physical and metaphorical foundation for forgiveness to occur, while forgiveness, in turn, opens up the space for deeper emotional healing and self-growth.

52. GROUNDING AND THE POWER OF GRATITUDE

Discussing the Benefits of Practicing Gratitude in Conjunction with Grounding Practices

Grounding and gratitude are two separate yet interconnected practices, each with their unique contributions to overall wellbeing. Grounding involves physical connection with the earth's surface to harness its natural energy, while gratitude is the conscious act of appreciating and giving thanks for the positive aspects of life. Integrating these two practices can provide a powerful framework for personal growth, emotional balance, and a deeper connection to the natural world.

The Power of Gratitude

Gratitude is a potent emotional and mental practice that shifts our focus from what we lack to the abundance that already exists in our lives. Regularly expressing gratitude can improve our mental health, strengthen our relationships, and even enhance our physical wellbeing.

Research has shown that gratitude can increase happiness, reduce depression, and improve resilience in the face of adversity. It encourages a positive outlook, fostering a greater appreciation for life's simple pleasures and a more profound connection to the world around us.

Interweaving Grounding and Gratitude

By marrying grounding and gratitude practices, we can deepen our relationship with ourselves and the natural world. Grounding in nature inherently lends itself to a state of gratitude. As we feel the earth beneath our feet, listen to the rustling leaves, or watch the waves lap against the shore, it's hard not to feel a sense of awe and appreciation for the natural world.

While grounded, we can intentionally cultivate a state of gratitude, perhaps by expressing thanks for the healing energy of the earth, the beauty of nature, or the very sensation of the ground beneath us. This can enrich our grounding practice, making it not just a physical experience but an emotional and spiritual one too.

Practical Techniques for Grounding and Gratitude

Grounding Gratitude Meditation: While sitting or lying outdoors, focus on the sensation of connection with the earth. Begin a gratitude meditation by mentally listing things you are grateful for, starting with the immediate sensations provided by the grounding experience.

Gratitude Walks: Walking barefoot outdoors combines physical grounding with the opportunity for mindful gratitude. As you walk, acknowledge your gratitude for each aspect of nature you encounter.

Gratitude Journaling in Nature: Bring your journal outdoors and find a comfortable spot to ground yourself. As you write down things you're grateful for, allow the connection to the earth to inspire your entries.

Mindful Gardening: Gardening is a naturally grounding activity. As you plant, weed, or prune, consciously express gratitude for the earth's fertility and the cycle of growth and renewal.

The Synergistic Effect of Grounding and Gratitude

The integration of grounding and gratitude creates a powerful synergy for wellbeing. Grounding allows us to draw upon the earth's healing energy, reducing physical and emotional discomfort, and promoting a sense of calm. Adding the practice of gratitude to this experience amplifies its benefits, helping us foster a positive outlook and a deeper appreciation for our connection to the natural world.

CONCLUSION

Grounding and gratitude, as separate practices, offer significant benefits for our mental, emotional, and physical health. When combined, these benefits can be significantly amplified, providing a pathway to enhanced wellbeing and a richer, more profound experience of life.

As we physically connect with the earth and consciously cultivate a state of gratitude, we can begin to perceive our world from a place of abundance, rather than lack. This shift in perspective, powered by the combined practices of grounding and gratitude, has the potential to lead to a profound transformation in our health, happiness, and overall quality of life.

53. GROUNDING AND THE POWER OF CONNECTION

Investigating how Grounding practices can foster a deeper sense of connection with oneself, others, and the environment.

Grounding and the Power of Connection: Investigating how Grounding Practices Can Foster a Deeper Sense of Connection with Oneself, Others, and the Environment

In our fast-paced, technologically-driven world, feeling disconnected – from ourselves, from each other, and from the environment – can be all too common. Grounding, a practice rooted in the reconnection to Earth's natural energies, offers a powerful antidote. By integrating grounding practices into our daily lives, we can cultivate a deeper sense of connection, not just with ourselves, but also with others and the environment.

Grounding: A Primer

Beyond the physical benefits, grounding has a profound impact on our mental and emotional health. It promotes calmness, reduces stress, improves focus and attention, and engenders a deep sense of connectedness that extends to our relationships and the environment.

Connection to Self

Grounding is an intrinsically mindful practice. As we feel the texture of the Earth under our feet or the cool grass between our fingers, we are drawn into the present moment, which helps anchor us in self-awareness and mindfulness.

Such mindful grounding exercises facilitate a deep connection to the self. We start to notice the subtleties of our bodily sensations, the ebb and flow of our emotions, and the patterns of our thoughts. This awareness helps us better understand our needs, desires, and boundaries, thereby nurturing self-compassion and self-respect.

Connection to Others

Human beings are social creatures; we thrive on connection and community. Grounding can foster a greater sense of connection to others, enhancing our relationships and interpersonal dynamics.

Firstly, the mental and emotional balance grounding promotes can make us more present in our interactions with others. This presence allows us to engage more authentically and meaningfully, fostering deeper relationships.

Secondly, grounding practices such as group meditations, barefoot walks, or grounding yoga classes, can serve as shared experiences, creating a sense of community and collective belonging.

Connection to the Environment

Grounding inherently connects us to the natural world. Feeling the Earth beneath us and the open sky above, we become attuned to the rhythms of nature. We're reminded that we're not separate entities, but part of a larger ecosystem.

This environmental connection engenders a deep respect and appreciation for nature, which can translate into more sustainable, eco-friendly habits. Additionally, research suggests that exposure to natural environments can reduce stress, improve mood, and enhance cognitive function, further attesting to the reciprocal relationship we share with the environment.

Cultivating Connection through Grounding: Practical Techniques

Barefoot Walks: Walking barefoot on natural ground is the simplest way to practice grounding. Pay attention to the sensations under your feet and the rhythm of your steps to enhance mindfulness.

Grounding Meditation: Find a quiet spot outdoors to sit or lie down directly on the ground. Tune into your breath and the sensations of the Earth beneath you.

Nature Immersion: Spend time in natural settings - forests, beaches, parks. Use all your senses to connect with your surroundings.

Group Grounding Activities: Participate in group activities that involve grounding, such as outdoor yoga classes or grounding workshops. Sharing the experience can deepen your sense of connection to others.

Conclusion

Grounding is more than just a therapeutic practice; it's a powerful conduit for connection. It encourages us to tune into ourselves, engage authentically with others, and appreciate the natural world that we are an intrinsic part of. By adopting regular grounding practices, we can counter the disconnection rampant in our modern lives, nurturing a profound sense of belonging and interconnectedness that contributes to our overall well-being. Grounding, in essence, reconnects us with the foundational elements of our existence, reminding us that at our core, we are intrinsically tied to the rhythms of the Earth and to one another.

54. GROUNDING AND THE POWER OF EMPATHY

Discussing How Grounding Practices Can Enhance Empathy and Compassion for Others

In our diverse and interconnected world, empathy and compassion are more crucial than ever. These are the skills that allow us to understand and resonate with the experiences of others, fostering genuine connection and promoting cooperation. Grounding, a practice that cultivates inner harmony by reconnecting us with the Earth, can significantly enhance our capacity for empathy and compassion. This essay delves into the intrinsic link between grounding practices and empathy and offers practical ways to harness this connection.

Understanding Grounding and Empathy

To comprehend the correlation between grounding and empathy, we need to understand the concepts themselves. Grounding, or earthing, is the practice of connecting physically with the Earth's surface – typically through barefoot contact with grass, sand, or dirt. This connection allows us to absorb the Earth's natural energy, which can result in a myriad of benefits, such as reduced stress and inflammation, improved mood, and increased overall wellbeing.

Empathy, on the other hand, is our ability to comprehend and share the feelings of others. It's about stepping into someone else's shoes and viewing the world from their perspective. Empathy, alongside compassion (the active desire to alleviate another's suffering), forms the backbone of positive social interaction and understanding.

The Grounding-Empathy Connection

Grounding's link to empathy lies in its influence on our emotional and mental states. Grounding is believed to facilitate the alignment of our bioenergetic field with that of the Earth. This alignment can foster a sense of calm, balance, and presence – key conditions for empathy to thrive.

When we're present and attuned to ourselves, we're better equipped to tune into others, fostering empathetic understanding. Grounding also promotes emotional resilience, allowing us to safely navigate our feelings and those of others without becoming overwhelmed.

How Grounding Enhances Empathy: The Science

Recent research has started to unravel the science behind grounding's empathetic benefits. Grounding appears to influence our autonomic nervous system (ANS), responsible for controlling our body's unconscious functions, including heart rate and stress response. By moderating the ANS, grounding can reduce anxiety and foster calm, thereby making empathy more accessible.

Grounding has also been associated with changes in brain wave patterns, shifting towards alpha and theta states, often linked to relaxation, creativity, and heightened emotional awareness – traits beneficial for empathy.

Practical Grounding Techniques to Boost Empathy

Barefoot Grounding: Simply walk barefoot on grass, sand, or soil. This direct contact allows you to absorb the Earth's natural energy, fostering emotional balance and presence.

Grounding Meditation: Sit or lie directly on the ground outdoors and focus on the sensations of the Earth beneath you. This can enhance mindfulness and openness to others' experiences.

Grounding Yoga: Incorporate grounding yoga poses such as Mountain Pose or Tree Pose. Performing these barefoot on natural ground can help you feel more connected and empathetic.

Mindful Nature Walks: Engage all your senses while walking in a natural environment. The immersion in nature and grounding can boost empathy.

Fostering Empathy through Grounding: A Community Perspective

Collective grounding activities, like group meditations or grounding retreats, offer a powerful way to foster empathy. Shared experiences can promote understanding and strengthen connections, thereby nurturing empathetic relationships. Moreover, grounding in diverse natural environments can enhance appreciation for the planet, fostering empathy towards broader ecological issues.

Conclusion

In a world where division and misunderstanding can be all too common, empathy and compassion are our bridge to understanding and unity. Grounding practices offer a valuable tool to enhance these critical skills, fostering not only personal well-being but also healthier, more empathetic communities. As we deepen our connection to the Earth and ourselves, we naturally open ourselves to better understand and connect with others. Grounding, therefore, is not only a journey inward but also a pathway leading us towards greater connection and understanding of the world around us.

55. GROUNDING AND THE POWER OF BOUNDARIES

Exploring How Grounding Practices Can Support the Development of Healthy Boundaries and Self-Care

In our interconnected and fast-paced world, establishing and maintaining personal boundaries has become an increasingly necessary skill for maintaining a sense of self, achieving a healthy work-life balance, and cultivating well-being. Grounding, the practice of physically and emotionally connecting with the Earth, has profound implications for the establishment of these boundaries. In this essay, we will delve into the interplay between grounding practices, boundary-setting, and self-care, offering actionable insights for integrating grounding into personal boundary work.

Understanding Grounding, Boundaries, and Self-Care

At its core, grounding is the practice of fostering a sense of connection with the Earth, often achieved through physical contact with the ground. This practice has been linked to numerous health benefits, including reduced stress, improved mood, and enhanced physical well-being.

Boundaries, on the other hand, are the mental, emotional, and physical limits we establish to protect ourselves from being manipulated, used, or violated by others. They delineate where we end and where others begin and help us maintain a healthy sense of self-respect and personal identity.

Self-care involves the actions we take to promote our own physical, emotional, and mental health. It requires an understanding of our own needs and making a commitment to meet them.

The Connection Between Grounding and Boundary Setting

The relationship between grounding and boundary setting lies in grounding's capacity to cultivate self-awareness, presence, and assertiveness—key components of healthy boundary setting. Grounding exercises help us tune into our physical and emotional experiences, fostering a deep sense of self-awareness. This awareness, coupled with the calm and focus derived from grounding, allows us to better identify our needs, recognize when they are not being met, and communicate these needs effectively to others.

Additionally, grounding can help us manage the emotional distress that often arises when setting or maintaining boundaries. By calming our nervous system and promoting a sense of safety, grounding can help us navigate these situations with greater ease and resilience.

How Grounding Supports Self-Care

Just as grounding enhances boundary setting, it also promotes self-care. Grounding practices inherently involve taking time to connect with oneself and the natural world, providing a respite from the demands of daily life and the constant stimuli of our digital world. This practice can be a form of self-care, helping to reduce stress and promote mental and physical well-being.

Moreover, by enhancing self-awareness and emotional regulation, grounding supports the ability to identify and respond to personal needs, laying the foundation for effective self-care strategies.

Practical Grounding Techniques to Support Boundaries and Self-Care

Barefoot Grounding: Walking barefoot on grass, sand, or soil can help you connect directly with the Earth's energy, promoting calmness, clarity, and resilience.

Grounding Meditation: Grounding meditations can help cultivate a strong sense of presence, fostering self-awareness and assertiveness, key elements of boundary setting.

Nature Immersion: Immersing yourself in nature, such as through forest bathing or gardening, can offer a restorative experience that promotes self-care and helps you feel grounded.

Grounding Visualizations: Visualization exercises, like imagining roots extending from your feet into the ground, can help strengthen your grounding practice and facilitate boundary work.

A Holistic Approach: Grounding, Boundaries, and Self-Care

Incorporating grounding practices into a holistic approach to setting boundaries and self-care can have transformative effects. This includes setting aside regular time for grounding activities, honoring your needs during these practices, and applying the self-awareness and resilience gained from grounding to boundary setting in your daily life.

Conclusion

In a world that constantly pushes us towards overextension, the practice of grounding offers a potent counterbalance, providing us with the tools to assert our boundaries and prioritize self-care. As we foster our connection to the Earth and ourselves, we naturally develop a greater understanding of our needs and the boundaries necessary to protect them. Thus, grounding practices offer an avenue not only for personal growth and well-being but also for the preservation and assertion of our unique identities in a demanding world.

56. GROUNDING AND THE POWER OF CREATIVITY

Investigating how Grounding Practices can Enhance Creativity and Artistic Expression

Creativity is a profound aspect of human experience. It is a vehicle for innovation, a catalyst for artistic expression, and a cornerstone of our ability to adapt to changing circumstances. In parallel, grounding practices, centered around forming a physical and spiritual connection to the Earth, are increasingly recognized for their potential to improve various aspects of well-being, including mental clarity, emotional stability, and physical health. In this exploration, we shall delve into how grounding practices may enhance creativity and inspire artistic expression, weaving together findings from scientific research, insights from artists and creators, and practical strategies for harnessing the potential synergies between these two potent forces.

Grounding and Creativity: The Connection

Grounding, or earthing, is a holistic practice focused on reconnecting individuals with the Earth's energy, usually achieved through direct physical contact with the ground. The process fosters a deep sense of calmness, connectedness, and balance, both mentally and physically.

Creativity, on the other hand, is an intricate process involving the generation of new ideas, solutions, or artistic expressions. It involves several cognitive processes, including divergent thinking (the ability to generate numerous ideas), convergent thinking (the ability to find the single best solution to a problem), and imaginative thought.

The intersection between grounding and creativity lies within their shared capacity to promote mental clarity, reduce stress, and foster a connection with our inner selves and the world around us. Grounding techniques, like walking barefoot on the ground, meditating in nature, or gardening, can help quiet the mind, allowing us to be more open and receptive to new ideas and perspectives. This mental calm and clarity can create an environment conducive to the flow of creativity.

Scientific Insights on Grounding and Creativity

Several studies have started to shed light on how grounding may indirectly influence creativity. Grounding has been associated with reducing inflammation, improving sleep, and lowering stress levels. All these factors can contribute to an optimal brain state for creativity. When we're relaxed, well-rested, and free from worry, our minds are more able to generate creative thoughts and ideas.

Furthermore, grounding practices often involve spending time in natural settings, which has its own set of creative benefits. Research has shown that exposure to nature can boost mood, enhance cognition, and spark creativity. Nature's sights, sounds, and smells can stimulate the senses, providing a rich source of inspiration for creative work.

Grounding Practices to Enhance Creativity

Barefoot Grounding: Walking barefoot on natural surfaces like grass, sand, or soil can help establish a direct connection with the

Earth. This practice can calm the mind and body, potentially leading to increased creative thinking.

Nature Meditation: Practicing meditation in natural settings can further enhance the grounding experience. By focusing on the sounds, smells, and sensations of nature during meditation, individuals can foster a deeper sense of presence and openness to creative inspiration.

Gardening: Engaging with the Earth directly, as in gardening, can be a form of grounding. This activity allows for creative expression while maintaining a physical connection with the Earth.

Nature Art: Creating art in or inspired by nature can help channel the grounding experience into artistic expression. Whether through painting, photography, or writing, nature can serve as a catalyst for creativity.

Grounding, Creativity, and Artistic Expression: A Synergistic Trio

Incorporating grounding practices into a creative routine can be a potent strategy for artists, innovators, and anyone seeking to boost their creative capabilities. By grounding themselves, individuals can create a mental and emotional state conducive to the flow of creativity. This synergy can enhance not only the quantity of creative output but also the depth and authenticity of the creative expression.

Conclusion

Grounding, with its calming, balancing effects, offers a unique pathway to enhance creativity and deepen artistic expression. By cultivating a physical and emotional connection to the Earth, grounding can help quiet the mind, providing a fertile ground for the seeds of creativity to take root and flourish. As we continue to explore the interplay between grounding and creativity, we can look forward to harnessing these practices' combined power to enhance our creative lives and, by extension, our overall well-being.

57. GROUNDING AND THE POWER OF MOVEMENT

Discussing the Benefits of Incorporating Movement and Physical Activity into Grounding Practices

Movement is fundamental to human life. It is our primary means of interacting with the world around us and an essential ingredient in our overall well-being. Movement, in the form of physical activity, not only keeps our bodies healthy but also promotes mental health by regulating mood and reducing stress. Grounding, on the other hand, is a practice that encourages a direct connection with the Earth's energy, often through physical contact with the ground, to promote health and well-being. But what happens when these two practices intertwine? This discussion explores the integration of movement into grounding practices and how this combination can enhance the benefits of each, leading to heightened physical health, mental clarity, and spiritual connection.

Grounding and Movement: A Natural Pair

Grounding and movement are intrinsically linked. Grounding often involves bodily contact with the Earth, typically through the soles of the feet, while movement involves the locomotion of the body. The fusion of these two practices involves activities that encourage both movement and direct contact with the Earth's surface. These activities can range from grounding yoga practices and earthing barefoot walks to dynamic meditation exercises carried out in nature.

The Benefits of Grounding and Movement

The benefits of grounding and movement are multidimensional, offering physical, mental, and spiritual gains.

Physical Benefits: Research has suggested that grounding can reduce inflammation, improve sleep, and support the body's healing processes. Movement, on the other hand, is well-known for its physical benefits, such as enhancing cardiovascular health, improving strength and flexibility, and promoting weight management. When combined, grounding and movement can synergistically promote physical well-being.

Mental Benefits: Grounding and movement both offer significant mental health benefits. Grounding can help reduce stress and anxiety, promote better sleep, and enhance focus and concentration. Movement is known to release endorphins, the body's natural mood lifters, and is used as a practical strategy in managing mental health conditions such as depression and anxiety. Together, grounding and movement can contribute to enhanced mental clarity and emotional stability.

Spiritual Benefits: Grounding, by nature, encourages a deeper connection with the Earth and the energy it exudes, fostering a sense of interconnectedness with nature and the wider universe. Movement, especially when intentional and mindful, can be a form of moving meditation, facilitating spiritual exploration and growth. When combined, grounding and movement can promote a greater sense of presence, heighten awareness, and deepen spiritual connection.

Incorporating Movement into Grounding Practices

There are several ways to incorporate movement into grounding practices.

Barefoot Walks or Runs: Walking or running barefoot on natural surfaces such as grass, sand, or dirt can connect us with the Earth's energy while promoting physical activity.

Grounding Yoga: Performing yoga poses barefoot on the ground, especially in a natural environment, combines the grounding effects of direct contact with the Earth with the mind-body benefits of yoga.

Outdoor Dance or Movement Classes: Participating in outdoor dance or movement classes encourages both grounding and physical activity. Dance forms like Qigong or Tai Chi that emphasize flowing movements and deep connections to nature are excellent options.

Dynamic Grounding Exercises: These are exercises designed to enhance grounding while incorporating movement, such as hopping or jumping barefoot on the ground or walking in patterns like figure eights.

Conclusion

Incorporating movement into grounding practices provides a potent strategy to enhance physical health, promote mental clarity, and deepen spiritual connection. The amalgamation of these practices encourages a heightened sense of overall well-being, balancing the energies within and around us. As we become more aware of our bodies in motion and more in tune with the energy of the Earth beneath us, we foster a deeper, more meaningful connection to ourselves, to nature, and to the rhythms of life.

58. GROUNDING AND THE POWER OF NUTRITION

Exploring How Grounding Practices Can Be Complemented by a Healthy and Nourishing Diet

The synergy of grounding and nutrition forms a strong foundation for holistic health and well-being. Grounding or earthing is a practice of direct contact with the Earth's surface, aligning the body with the natural electric charge present in the Earth. This practice helps to stabilize the body's internal bioelectrical environment and can offer numerous health benefits. On the other hand, nutrition focuses on consuming a balanced diet that supplies essential nutrients to the body for optimal functioning. Merging these two practices can result in a powerful, synergistic effect, maximizing the potential benefits of both.

Grounding: A Foundation for Health

Grounding is increasingly recognized for its potential benefits. Studies suggest that this simple practice can reduce inflammation, enhance sleep, improve wound healing, and promote overall well-being. The principle behind these benefits is the flow of electrons from the Earth into the body, which may neutralize harmful free radicals and reduce oxidative stress. Grounding also aids in balancing the autonomic nervous system and enhancing heart rate variability, reflecting improved stress response and vitality.

The Power of Nutrition

Proper nutrition is pivotal for overall health and wellbeing. Consuming a diet rich in a variety of fruits, vegetables, whole grains, lean proteins, and healthy fats can provide the body with essential nutrients. These nutrients are the building blocks of health, vital for growth, disease prevention, energy production, and the maintenance of body functions. Nutrient-dense foods also provide antioxidants, similar to grounding, which combat oxidative stress and reduce inflammation. Nutrition and grounding can therefore act in concert, offering a powerful tool for health promotion.

Symbiosis of Grounding and Nutrition

The interplay between grounding and nutrition can be particularly potent. Both practices enhance the body's capacity to heal and regenerate, acting as powerful allies in the quest for health and longevity. Here are some ways these practices can complement each other:

Reduced Inflammation: Both grounding and a nutrient-rich diet can help reduce inflammation. Grounding is believed to neutralize free radicals and reduce inflammation through the influx of negatively charged electrons from the Earth. A diet rich in antioxidants from fruits, vegetables, and other whole foods also combats inflammation, assisting the body's natural defenses.

Enhanced Healing: Grounding may enhance wound healing by optimizing the body's bioelectrical environment. Nutrition also plays a critical role in healing, as nutrients such as protein, vitamins A and C, and zinc are essential for wound repair and tissue growth.

Improved Sleep and Relaxation: Grounding can help improve sleep and promote relaxation by influencing the autonomic nervous system and cortisol production. Certain nutrients, like magnesium and tryptophan, found in foods like leafy greens and turkey, can also promote better sleep and relaxation.

Boosted Immunity: Grounding and a healthy diet can both support the immune system. Grounding enhances overall wellbeing and reduces stress, which can bolster immune function. Meanwhile, many nutrients, such as vitamins A, C, D, and E, and minerals like zinc and selenium, are vital for maintaining a strong immune system.

Integrating Grounding and Nutrition into Daily Life

Creating a routine that incorporates both grounding and nutrition can be relatively straightforward. Begin by setting aside daily time for grounding. This could be walking barefoot in the grass, meditating outdoors, gardening, or even swimming in natural bodies of water. Then, ensure your diet is rich in a variety of whole foods, emphasizing fruits, vegetables, whole grains, lean proteins, and healthy fats. Strive to consume a rainbow of fruits and vegetables to maximize antioxidant intake, and prioritize unprocessed foods whenever possible.

Conclusion

Grounding and nutrition are both potent tools for health promotion. By integrating these practices into daily life, individuals can tap into a powerful synergy that supports reduced inflammation, enhanced healing, improved sleep and relaxation, and boosted immunity. As our understanding of these practices continues to deepen, the combination of grounding and nutrition offers a promising avenue for enhancing health and wellbeing. This harmonious approach not only nurtures the body but also fosters a deeper connection with our environment, reminding us of the vital role our planet plays in our health.

59. GROUNDING AND THE POWER OF MINDFUL EATING

Investigating How Mindful Eating Practices Can Enhance the Grounding Experience and Promote Overall Health

Grounding and mindful eating are two potent practices that intertwine to foster a holistic approach to health and well-being. Grounding, also known as earthing, is the process of connecting directly with the Earth's surface, facilitating a flow of electrons that can help neutralize free radicals and reduce inflammation. Mindful eating, on the other hand, is a conscious practice of being fully aware of the food we consume and the process of eating, leading to improved eating behaviors, digestion, and overall health. These two practices can harmoniously blend, creating a nourishing environment for both the body and mind.

Grounding: The Power of Earth Connection

The art of grounding or earthing roots in the fundamental principle of achieving an electrical balance within our bodies through direct contact with the Earth. This connection helps to regulate our internal bioelectrical environment, reduce inflammation, improve sleep, and enhance general well-being. As modern lifestyles often involve spending significant time indoors and away from natural environments, grounding offers an easy and natural way to reconnect with the Earth and our natural rhythms.

Mindful Eating: The Power of Presence

Mindful eating is a practice that encourages an individual to pay full attention to the experience of eating and drinking, both inside and outside the body. This awareness includes recognizing the colors, smells, flavors, textures, and temperatures of our food, observing the body's hunger and satiety cues, and acknowledging the interconnection between the Earth, our food, and our health. Mindful eating is not just about eating slowly or without distraction, but also about understanding the nutritional and energetic content of food and recognizing the impact of our food choices on our body and the environment.

Interplay Between Grounding and Mindful Eating

Grounding and mindful eating are integrative practices that can enhance one another, creating a powerful synergy that supports overall health and well-being. Here's how:

Awareness and Connection: Both grounding and mindful eating promote a greater awareness of our bodies and our connection with the environment. Grounding allows us to experience the Earth's energy directly, while mindful eating encourages us to consider where our food comes from and how it affects our bodies.

Reducing Stress and Inflammation: Grounding has been shown to reduce stress and inflammation, as does mindful eating. By slowing down and savoring our meals, we can reduce overeating and the associated inflammation caused by poor dietary choices.

Promoting Satiety and Digestive Health: Mindful eating can help us recognize when we're full, reducing the likelihood of overeating. Grounding, particularly when practiced outdoors during meal times, can further enhance this awareness by providing a calming environment conducive to slow, mindful eating.

Environmental Consideration: Both practices encourage a greater appreciation for our environment. Grounding fosters a tangible connection to the Earth, while mindful eating can make us more aware of the environmental impact of our food choices, encouraging more sustainable practices.

Integrating Grounding and Mindful Eating into Daily Life

Integrating grounding and mindful eating into daily life can be a seamless process. Begin by setting aside specific times to practice grounding, like early morning or late afternoon. This could involve walking barefoot in a park or simply standing barefoot on the ground. For mindful eating, start by eliminating distractions during meal times. Focus on the smell, taste, and texture of your food, and pay attention to your hunger and fullness cues. Over time, you could also consider integrating these practices, perhaps by eating meals outdoors barefoot when possible.

Conclusion

The synergy between grounding and mindful eating provides a powerful approach to health and wellness. By combining these practices, we can develop a deeper understanding of our bodies, our food, and our connection with the Earth, ultimately promoting a healthier, more mindful lifestyle. As we continue to navigate through our fast-paced world, these practices offer a refuge - a way to slow down, reconnect with our natural rhythms, and cultivate a profound sense of awareness and appreciation for our health and our planet.

60. GROUNDING AND THE POWER OF MINDFUL COMMUNICATION

Discussing How Grounding Practices Can Support Mindful Communication and Enhance Relationships

In the modern, fast-paced world, authentic and thoughtful communication often becomes sidelined. We live in an era of multitasking and digital distractions, where mindful communication — the practice of being present, attentive, and open in our interactions with others — is more of a luxury than the norm. Grounding, a practice rooted in connection with the Earth and self, offers a route to rejuvenate our communication skills, enhance our relationships, and strengthen our bonds with others.

Beyond physical benefits, grounding can have a profound impact on our emotional and mental well-being. It instills a sense of calm, presence, and awareness that allows us to be more in tune with our thoughts, feelings, and reactions — vital elements for mindful communication.

Mindful Communication: The Heart of Relationships

Mindful communication is a conscious, deliberate way of communicating, where one remains fully present, listens attentively, and speaks truthfully. It encourages empathy, understanding, and deep, meaningful connections. Mindful communication goes beyond the spoken words; it involves understanding the underlying feelings and emotions, thereby leading to an enriched, fulfilling, and respectful exchange.

The Connection between Grounding and Mindful Communication

Grounding can pave the way for more mindful communication in a number of ways.

Promoting Presence and Awareness: Grounding fosters a state of mindfulness, bringing us into the present moment. This heightened awareness can significantly enhance our communication skills, as it allows us to fully engage in conversations, attentively listen, and respond thoughtfully.

Managing Emotional Reactivity: Grounding can help manage emotional reactivity, reducing the likelihood of reactive and heated conversations. It provides a calming effect, helping us to stay balanced even in emotionally charged situations, enabling more thoughtful and compassionate responses.

Enhancing Empathy and Connection: As grounding connects us to nature and to ourselves, it also fosters a sense of connection with others. This interconnectedness promotes empathy — the ability to understand and share the feelings of others — which is a key aspect of mindful communication.

Facilitating Authenticity and Openness: Grounding can help us to connect deeply with our true selves, fostering authenticity in our interactions. This openness allows for more honest and meaningful exchanges, enhancing the quality of our relationships.

Integrating Grounding and Mindful Communication into Daily Life

Bringing grounding and mindful communication into daily practice is simple yet transformative. Regularly spending time in nature, walking barefoot, or even simply connecting with the Earth physically in any way possible can make a significant difference to one's sense of grounding.

Mindful communication, on the other hand, requires conscious practice. Start by simply being present in conversations, actively listening without planning your response, acknowledging the other person's feelings, and speaking from a place of compassion and understanding. Combining these practices — grounding yourself before or during discussions — can contribute greatly to the quality of your communications.

Conclusion

The intersection of grounding and mindful communication presents a unique avenue to elevate our relationships. As we ground ourselves, we become more present, less reactive, and more connected — all of which foster genuine, mindful communication. As we continue to navigate the challenges of modern living, these practices offer us a way to enhance our relationships, connect on a deeper level, and ultimately enrich our life experience.

61. GROUNDING AND THE POWER OF MINDFUL PARENTING

Exploring How Grounding Practices Can Support Mindful Parenting and Enhance Family Relationships

In an increasingly complex and fast-paced world, parents often feel overwhelmed by the pressures of raising children. The practice of mindful parenting, which incorporates principles of mindfulness into parenting, offers a potential solution to this challenge. Simultaneously, grounding, a holistic practice of reconnecting with the Earth's energy, can offer complementary benefits. Together, mindful parenting and grounding can enhance family relationships, creating an environment of empathy, understanding, and tranquility.

The Concept of Grounding and Its Potential Benefits

Grounding, also known as Earthing, is the practice of establishing a direct connection with the Earth's surface. Whether through walking barefoot on grass or sitting on the beach, grounding connects us to the Earth's natural electric charge. Advocates of grounding believe it helps balance our bioelectrical environment, resulting in various physical benefits like reduced inflammation, stress relief, improved sleep, and enhanced immune responses.

The psychological benefits of grounding are equally potent. It fosters mindfulness, enhances our connection to nature, and promotes emotional regulation and tranquility, all of which can indirectly contribute to improved parent-child relationships.

Understanding Mindful Parenting

Mindful parenting involves applying mindfulness principles — presence, acceptance, and nonjudgmental awareness — to the parenting process. It invites parents to respond rather than react to parenting situations, deeply understand their child's needs, and cultivate a nonjudgmental and compassionate family environment.

Mindful parenting has been linked with numerous positive outcomes, including reduced parental stress, enhanced parental satisfaction, and improved child behavior and mental health.

The Intersection of Grounding and Mindful Parenting

Grounding can significantly contribute to mindful parenting by offering several key benefits:

Fostering Presence and Awareness: By centering our focus on the physical connection with the Earth, grounding brings us into the present moment. This presence can be incredibly beneficial for mindful parenting, allowing parents to engage fully with their children, without distraction.

Promoting Emotional Regulation: Grounding's calming influence can help manage emotional reactivity, a common challenge in parenting. By fostering inner peace and tranquility, grounding allows parents to approach challenging situations with calmness and clarity.

Cultivating Empathy and Connection: As grounding deepens our connection to the Earth and ourselves, it simultaneously enhances our connection with others, fostering empathy. This can translate to greater understanding and compassion in parent-child interactions.

Enhancing Resilience: The combination of grounding and mindful parenting can also help families to foster resilience. By teaching children to remain connected and present, even during challenging times, these practices can equip them with essential life skills.

Integrating Grounding and Mindful Parenting Into Daily Life

Incorporating grounding and mindful parenting into daily life can be relatively straightforward. Families can introduce grounding through regular activities such as walks in the park, gardening, or picnics on the beach. By consciously engaging in these activities without digital distractions, parents can model mindful behavior and encourage their children to adopt similar practices.

Mindful parenting can be practiced by maintaining an open and accepting attitude towards parenting challenges, listening empathetically to children's concerns, and being fully present in shared moments.

Conclusion

When integrated thoughtfully, grounding and mindful parenting can enhance familial relationships and contribute to a harmonious family environment. These practices offer an invaluable resource for parents seeking to navigate the complexities of modern family life. By fostering presence, empathy, and emotional regulation, grounding and mindful parenting hold the potential to nurture deeper parent-child connections and create a resilient, compassionate, and mindful family unit.

62. GROUNDING AND THE POWER OF MINDFUL LEADERSHIP

Investigating How Grounding Practices Can Support Mindful Leadership and Enhance Workplace Culture

Today's fast-paced, high-stress corporate landscape often fuels a culture of burnout, contributing to low morale, poor productivity, and frequent turnover. In response to this challenge, many leaders are turning to mindful leadership — a leadership style grounded in mindfulness and presence — to promote a healthier, more resilient, and more productive work environment. Further, grounding, the practice of connecting with the Earth's energy, can supplement this mindful leadership approach, offering numerous potential benefits for leaders and their teams.

Understanding Grounding and Its Benefits

Grounding, also known as earthing, refers to the practice of physically connecting with the Earth — walking barefoot on grass, for example — to tap into the planet's natural energy. Grounding advocates assert that this practice provides a myriad of benefits, ranging from reduced inflammation and stress levels to improved sleep and immunity.

Beyond physical wellness, grounding can also cultivate psychological and emotional wellbeing. It fosters mindfulness, encourages a connection with nature, and promotes emotional regulation and tranquility, crucial elements that can contribute to more effective leadership.

The Concept of Mindful Leadership

Mindful leadership revolves around the application of mindfulness principles — presence, awareness, and nonjudgmental acceptance — to leadership roles. A mindful leader is one who can remain calm under pressure, listen deeply, communicate effectively, and make thoughtful decisions.

By encouraging responsiveness rather than reactivity, mindful leadership can lead to improved team morale, enhanced productivity, better decision-making, and a more innovative and resilient work culture.

The Intersection of Grounding and Mindful Leadership

The integration of grounding practices into mindful leadership can provide several important benefits.

Promotes Presence and Awareness: Grounding can help leaders become more present and aware, essential characteristics of mindful leadership. By focusing on the physical connection with the Earth, grounding brings us into the present moment, reducing distractions and encouraging full engagement.

Enhances Emotional Regulation: Grounding practices can help manage emotional reactivity, a common challenge in high-pressure leadership roles. The calming influence of grounding can equip leaders with a tranquil mindset, allowing them to approach challenging situations with calmness and clarity.

Fosters Empathy and Connection: Grounding enhances our connection with the Earth and ourselves, and by extension, with others. This can result in increased empathy and understanding, fostering better leader-team relationships and more effective communication.

Encourages Resilience: By combining grounding and mindful leadership, organizations can cultivate resilience. Grounding teaches leaders to stay connected and present, even under pressure, equipping them and their teams with essential stress management tools.

Integrating Grounding and Mindful Leadership in the Workplace

Incorporating grounding and mindful leadership practices in the workplace can take various forms. Organizations might consider instituting regular outdoor team-building activities, encouraging break times spent in natural settings, or even just advocating for employees to spend some of their off-hours outdoors. Leaders can model these behaviors, setting a precedent for their teams.

Mindful leadership can be practiced by maintaining an open, nonjudgmental approach to leadership challenges, actively listening to team members, and taking time for mindful reflection before decision-making.

Conclusion

The integration of grounding practices and mindful leadership can significantly enhance workplace culture, fostering a more empathetic, resilient, and productive work environment. As leaders become more present, emotionally regulated, and empathetic, teams become more connected, innovative, and resilient. In this way, the combination of grounding and mindful leadership offers a powerful strategy for addressing workplace stress and burnout and fostering a more mindful, balanced, and thriving work culture.

63. GROUNDING AND THE POWER OF MINDFUL TECHNOLOGY USE

Discussing How Grounding Practices Can Support Mindful Technology Use and Promote Digital Well-Being

In our hyper-connected world, digital technology pervades every aspect of our lives. However, alongside the numerous benefits of this connectivity, concerns about digital overuse and the impact on our health and well-being have risen. Consequently, mindful technology use, which encourages conscious and intentional engagement with technology, has become increasingly significant. Combining mindful technology use with grounding practices can provide a holistic approach to promote digital well-being.

Understanding Grounding and Its Potential Benefits

Grounding, often referred to as earthing, is a practice that involves connecting with the Earth's natural energy, typically by going barefoot on natural surfaces like grass or sand. Advocates of grounding highlight various potential benefits, including reduced inflammation, improved sleep, enhanced mood, and lower stress levels. Moreover, grounding can help reconnect us to nature, promote mindfulness, and foster a sense of tranquility and well-being.

Mindful Technology Use and Its Importance

Mindful technology use promotes an intentional and conscious engagement with our devices. Instead of mindlessly scrolling or succumbing to digital distractions, mindful technology use encourages us to ask ourselves: Why am I reaching for this device? What do I hope to gain from it? Is this the best use of my time?

Such mindful engagement helps to combat digital overload, reduces stress, and promotes healthier technology habits. It can enhance productivity, improve sleep, and reduce feelings of anxiety and depression linked to excessive screen time.

Combining Grounding Practices and Mindful Technology Use

Grounding and mindful technology use are not mutually exclusive; instead, they complement each other and can be combined effectively.

Promoting Digital Detoxes: Grounding provides an excellent opportunity for digital detoxes. Spending time outdoors, connected to the Earth, offers a break from screens, allowing the mind and eyes to rest.

Fostering Presence and Awareness: Grounding can enhance our awareness and presence, essential elements of mindful technology use. It helps us remain in the present moment, makes us more aware of our habits, and can provide a mental note to pause before reaching for a device impulsively.

Enhancing Emotional Regulation: Grounding can help manage our emotional state, making us less susceptible to digital distractions or online provocations. This emotional stability can lead to more mindful technology use.

Reconnecting with Nature: Grounding rekindles our connection with nature, providing a refreshing contrast to the digital world. This connection can remind us of the value of offline experiences and foster a healthier balance between digital and real-world engagement.

Practical Steps for Grounding and Mindful Technology Use

To integrate grounding and mindful technology use into daily life, consider the following strategies.

Create tech-free zones or times: Dedicate certain times or areas in your home where technology use is off-limits. Use this time for grounding practices like gardening or walking barefoot outdoors.

Practice grounding during breaks: Use breaks from technology to practice grounding. This practice can help clear your mind, reset your focus, and reduce the risk of digital fatigue.

Set clear intentions: Before reaching for your device, set a clear intention. Coupling this mindful practice with regular grounding can help foster more conscious technology use.

Regular digital detoxes: Schedule regular digital detoxes where you spend the entire day or weekend without technology, focusing instead on grounding and other offline activities.

Conclusion

In the digital age, grounding and mindful technology use can provide a balanced approach to digital well-being. By reconnecting with nature, promoting presence and awareness, and enhancing emotional regulation, we can navigate the digital world more mindfully. In essence, grounding practices offer a valuable counterpoint to our technology-filled lives, fostering a healthier relationship with our devices, enhancing our well-being, and creating a more mindful and balanced lifestyle.

64. GROUNDING AND THE POWER OF MINDFUL TRAVEL

Exploring How Grounding Practices Can Enhance Travel Experiences and Promote Cultural Awareness

Travel is often considered a catalyst for personal growth, perspective shifts, and a broader understanding of the world. The excitement of exploring new territories, experiencing different cultures, and immersing oneself in the unfamiliar can be transformational. However, as thrilling as these experiences can be, they can also be overwhelming, making it crucial to remain grounded. Grounding, paired with mindful travel, can significantly enhance the travel experience, deepen cultural awareness, and promote a more meaningful connection with the places visited and their inhabitants.

Understanding Grounding and Its Importance

Grounding, or earthing, is a practice rooted in the concept of reconnecting physically and spiritually with the Earth. It is a practice that involves activities such as walking barefoot on natural surfaces, meditating outdoors, or even just spending time in nature. Grounding can provide a sense of balance and calm, helping us to stay present and connected in a rapidly changing environment, such as when traveling.

Mindful Travel: An Overview

Mindful travel is about being present and fully engaged in the travel experience. It encourages travelers to slow down, to observe the world around them consciously, and to engage with their surroundings in a meaningful and respectful manner. Mindful travel can lead to deeper cultural understanding, stronger connections with locals, and a greater appreciation for the natural world.

How Grounding Practices Enhance Mindful Travel

Incorporating grounding practices into travel routines can provide several key benefits:

Promotes Presence and Engagement: Grounding helps travelers to stay present and connected to their experiences. It encourages a deeper awareness and appreciation of new environments, promoting active engagement rather than passive observation.

Offers Emotional Stability: Travel can be emotionally overwhelming, with new experiences, sights, and sounds bombarding the senses. Grounding helps maintain emotional balance, reducing stress, and anxiety, and making it easier to navigate unfamiliar environments.

Supports Physical Health: Travel can be physically demanding, with different time zones, diet changes, and long days of exploration. Grounding practices like walking barefoot on the beach or in the grass can help manage jet lag, promote better sleep, and boost energy levels.

Fosters Cultural Understanding: Grounding encourages travelers to slow down, facilitating more meaningful interactions with locals and a more profound understanding of cultural nuances.

Applying Grounding Practices During Travel

Implementing grounding practices while traveling can take many forms.

Nature Immersion: Make time to connect with the natural environment. This could be a walk in the park, a hike, a swim in the ocean, or simply sitting quietly in a beautiful outdoor setting.

Mindful Observation: Practice mindful observation of the environment, engaging all your senses. Notice the sounds, smells, tastes, sights, and textures around you.

Local Engagement: Engage with local communities. Attend local events or festivals, visit local markets, or try local foods. These experiences provide opportunities for grounding by connecting more deeply with the culture and people of the place.

Physical Grounding: Whenever possible, go barefoot to physically connect with the Earth. Whether it's on a sandy beach, a grassy park, or a forest trail, this direct contact with the Earth can have a grounding effect.

Mindful Activities: Incorporate mindful activities into your travel itinerary. This could be a yoga class, a meditation session, or a quiet time for journaling at the end of the day.

Conclusion

Travel offers a wealth of experiences that can enrich our lives in myriad ways. However, to fully appreciate and absorb these experiences, it's essential to remain grounded and present. By integrating grounding practices into our travel routines, we can enhance our travel experiences, deepen our understanding of the cultures we encounter, and cultivate a richer, more meaningful connection with the world around us. Ultimately, grounding, combined with mindful travel, offers a pathway to a more fulfilling and transformative journey.

65. GROUNDING AND THE POWER OF MINDFUL AGING

Investigating how Grounding practices can support healthy aging and promote longevity

Grounding and the Power of Mindful Aging: Investigating How Grounding Practices Can Support Healthy Aging and Promote Longevity.

Aging is an inevitable part of the human journey, and it is often associated with physical decline, mental deterioration, and a loss of independence. However, this narrative can be shifted by embracing a more positive and mindful approach towards aging. Grounding, also known as earthing, combined with mindful aging, can significantly enhance the quality of life, promote health and well-being, and potentially extend longevity.

Understanding Grounding and Its Benefits

Grounding is a therapeutic practice that connects individuals physically and energetically with the Earth. It involves activities such as walking barefoot on the grass, swimming in natural bodies of water, or simply spending time in nature. This connection to the Earth has been shown to have numerous health benefits, including reduced inflammation, improved sleep, and enhanced immunity – all of which are particularly beneficial for aging individuals.

What is Mindful Aging?

Mindful aging refers to the practice of fully embracing each moment of the aging process with presence, acceptance, and self-compassion. It involves acknowledging and accepting the changes that come with age, while also taking proactive steps to maintain physical health, mental acuity, and emotional well-being.

Grounding Practices for Mindful Aging

Integrating grounding practices into a mindful aging strategy can offer multiple benefits. Here's how:

Reduced Chronic Inflammation: Chronic inflammation is associated with various age-related diseases like arthritis, heart disease, and Alzheimer's. Research suggests that grounding can reduce inflammation by neutralizing free radicals in the body, potentially slowing the onset of these diseases and promoting healthier aging.

Enhanced Emotional Well-being: Spending time in nature and engaging in grounding practices can improve mood, reduce stress, and alleviate symptoms of depression and anxiety. This emotional stability is crucial in maintaining a positive outlook towards aging.

Greater Physical Mobility: Grounding activities, especially those involving gentle, physical movement like barefoot walking or gardening, can help maintain strength, flexibility, and balance – all important for maintaining mobility and independence in later years.

Practical Grounding Techniques for Healthy Aging

Grounding practices can be incorporated into daily routines in various ways.

Barefoot Walking: Taking regular walks barefoot in a safe, natural environment can help you connect directly with the Earth's energy. It's also an excellent opportunity for light exercise.

Grounding Meditation: Practicing meditation outdoors, sitting on the grass or the bare ground, can enhance your grounding practice while promoting relaxation and mental clarity.

Gardening: Gardening is a fantastic grounding activity that also offers the satisfaction of growing your own food or flowers.

Swimming in Natural Waters: Whenever possible, swimming in the sea, lakes, or rivers can be highly grounding and also offers the benefits of low-impact exercise.

Using Grounding Devices: For those who have limited access to natural environments, grounding devices such as grounding mats or sheets can provide similar benefits.

Conclusion

Aging doesn't need to be a journey of decline and deterioration. By adopting grounding practices and embracing mindful aging, older adults can create a life that is vibrant, meaningful, and full of health. By acknowledging and accepting the inevitable changes that come with aging, and taking proactive steps to stay physically, mentally, and emotionally healthy, one can not only add years to life but also life to years. Grounding offers an accessible, natural, and holistic pathway to a healthier and more fulfilling aging process.

66. GROUNDING AND ADDICTION RECOVER

Exploring the Potential Benefits of Grounding Practices for Individuals in Addiction Recovery

Addiction is a complex and multifaceted condition that impacts every aspect of a person's life, including their physical health, emotional well-being, relationships, and societal functioning. The road to recovery is often long and challenging, requiring a comprehensive approach that addresses not only addictive behavior but also the underlying emotional and psychological issues. Grounding, a holistic practice that involves connecting physically and energetically with the earth, could offer unique benefits to individuals on this healing journey.

Scientific studies suggest that grounding can help reduce inflammation, improve sleep, decrease stress, and enhance overall well-being. These effects are potentially achieved through the neutralization of free radicals and the regulation of the body's circadian rhythms.

Grounding and Addiction Recovery

The benefits of grounding can be particularly helpful for individuals in addiction recovery. Here's how:

Stress Reduction: Stress and emotional instability are common triggers for addictive behaviors. Grounding practices can help reduce stress and promote emotional stability by rebalancing the body's electrical energy and promoting a sense of calm and relaxation.

Improved Sleep: Disrupted sleep patterns are common among individuals recovering from addiction, and poor sleep can exacerbate cravings and other withdrawal symptoms. Grounding can help improve sleep quality by helping to regulate the body's circadian rhythms.

Enhanced Physical Health: Substance abuse takes a significant toll on the body. By reducing inflammation and supporting overall physical health, grounding can support the body's healing process during recovery.

Increased Mindfulness: Grounding practices require an individual to focus on the present moment and their physical connection to the earth, which can promote mindfulness. This heightened awareness of one's body and surroundings can support the development of healthier coping mechanisms and reduce the likelihood of relapse.

Implementing Grounding Practices in Addiction Recovery

There are several ways to incorporate grounding into a recovery program.

Barefoot Walking or Running: Walking or running barefoot on the grass, sand, or dirt can be a highly effective grounding technique. This practice can be integrated into daily routines, offering a natural and accessible form of grounding.

Outdoor Meditation or Yoga: Practicing meditation or yoga outdoors on the bare ground can amplify the grounding effect and support mental and emotional well-being.

Swimming in Natural Water: Swimming in the sea, a lake, or a river can also offer grounding benefits. The water's conductivity can enhance the grounding effect, and the physical activity can provide additional health benefits.

Gardening: Gardening involves direct contact with the earth, making it another excellent grounding activity. Gardening also offers the added benefits of physical activity and the satisfaction of nurturing growth.

Using Grounding Devices: For those who have limited access to outdoor spaces, grounding devices such as grounding mats, sheets, or patches can be used to achieve a similar effect. These devices can be used while sleeping or sitting, making grounding achievable for almost anyone, anywhere.

Conclusion

Grounding, with its stress-reducing, sleep-enhancing, and health-promoting benefits, offers a powerful tool for individuals in addiction recovery. While it is not a standalone treatment for addiction, grounding can complement traditional treatment approaches, including therapy and medication. By promoting physical well-being, emotional stability, and mindfulness, grounding can support individuals on their journey to recovery and help them build healthier, substance-free lives. As always, any new practices should be undertaken in consultation with healthcare professionals and integrated into a comprehensive treatment plan.

67. GROUNDING AND TRAUMA HEALING

Discussing how Grounding practices can support trauma healing and emotional regulation

Trauma, whether it be physical, emotional, or psychological, can profoundly affect an individual's well-being and life quality. People living with trauma often experience a host of debilitating symptoms, including flashbacks, nightmares, anxiety, depression, and difficulties in emotional regulation. While traditional therapeutic interventions like cognitive behavioral therapy (CBT) and eye movement desensitization and reprocessing (EMDR) are often employed to treat trauma, grounding practices can offer a complementary and holistic approach that could enhance healing outcomes.

Scientific studies on grounding suggest its potential in reducing inflammation, enhancing sleep, mitigating stress, and improving overall well-being. Grounding's ability to normalize the body's biological rhythms and neutralize free radicals may underpin these benefits.

Grounding and Trauma Healing

Grounding's inherent benefits can be especially valuable in the context of trauma healing.

Stress Reduction: Trauma survivors often grapple with chronic stress and anxiety. Grounding can help alleviate these symptoms by rebalancing the body's electrical energy and promoting relaxation and calmness.

Emotional Regulation: Grounding fosters a state of mindfulness, encouraging individuals to stay present and connected to their physical reality. This focus on the here and now can aid in emotional regulation, allowing trauma survivors to better manage overwhelming feelings and reduce dissociative symptoms.

Improved Sleep: Trauma can significantly disrupt sleep patterns, causing nightmares and insomnia. Grounding may enhance sleep quality by aiding in the regulation of circadian rhythms, fostering better rest and recovery.

Enhanced Physical Health: Trauma can have profound effects on physical health, triggering inflammatory responses and a host of related health issues. Grounding's anti-inflammatory effects can support the body's natural healing processes.

Implementing Grounding Practices in Trauma Healing

Grounding can be incorporated into trauma healing routines in several ways.

Barefoot Walking or Running: Encourage regular barefoot walks or runs on grass, sand, or soil. This direct contact with the Earth offers a straightforward way to practice grounding.

Outdoor Meditation or Yoga: Outdoor meditation or yoga sessions on the bare ground can enhance the grounding effect. These practices can also aid in stress reduction and emotional regulation.

Swimming in Natural Water: Natural bodies of water like the ocean, lakes, and rivers can serve as effective grounding platforms. Besides the physical activity benefits, the water's conductivity can enhance the grounding effect.

Gardening: Direct contact with the Earth through gardening can provide grounding benefits. Gardening also offers the satisfaction of nurturing growth and can serve as a mindful, therapeutic activity.

Using Grounding Devices: Grounding mats, sheets, or patches can be useful for individuals with limited access to outdoor spaces. These devices can replicate the grounding effect when used during sleep or sedentary activities.

Conclusion

In summary, grounding, with its calming, sleep-enhancing, and health-promoting effects, presents a viable complementary approach in trauma healing. It fosters physical well-being and emotional regulation, facilitating a better capacity to process traumatic experiences. While grounding isn't a standalone solution for trauma, it can amplify the effects of traditional therapeutic interventions. As always, it's advisable to incorporate new practices into an existing treatment plan under professional supervision. Through grounding, trauma survivors can find a pathway towards improved well-being and emotional resilience.

68. GROUNDING AND THE POWER OF MIND-BODY CONNECTION

Investigating How Grounding Practices Can Facilitate a Deeper Mind-Body Connection and Promote Overall Well-being

The concept of a mind-body connection has been central to healthcare philosophies worldwide for centuries. This principle maintains that our emotional, mental, social, and behavioral factors can directly affect our physical health and vice versa. One way this connection can be fostered and enhanced is through grounding, also known as earthing. Grounding is a practice that involves physical contact with the Earth's surface, connecting us to its vast supply of electrons, which have been found to have numerous health benefits. This essay will investigate how grounding can aid in establishing a profound mind-body connection, promoting overall well-being.

The Science of Grounding

Grounding practices, such as walking barefoot on the Earth or using conductive systems in our homes while sleeping or working, connect us to the Earth's negative electric charge. Several scientific studies suggest that these practices can reduce inflammation, improve sleep, regulate the circadian rhythm, and decrease stress levels. Grounding can also help normalize cortisol secretion, a primary stress hormone, thereby aligning us with the natural rhythms of the day.

Promoting a Mind-Body Connection

So how does grounding facilitate a deeper mind-body connection? Let's explore.

Increased Mindfulness: Grounding often involves spending time in nature and focusing on physical sensations, which can bring us into the present moment. This increased mindfulness fosters a stronger mind-body connection, as we become more aware of our physical presence and sensations.

Stress Reduction: The physical contact with the Earth's surface during grounding practices has been shown to reduce stress and anxiety. When our mental state is calm and centered, we're better able to recognize and respond to our body's signals, enhancing the mind-body connection.

Improved Physical Health: Grounding's anti-inflammatory and sleep-enhancing effects contribute to overall physical well-being. A healthier body can influence our mental state positively, further strengthening the mind-body connection.

Emotional Regulation: Grounding encourages us to anchor ourselves in the present moment, which can help manage overwhelming emotions. This emotional regulation links our mental and physical experiences, reinforcing the mind-body connection.

Incorporating Grounding into Daily Life

How can we implement grounding practices to foster a better mind-body connection? Here are some suggestions.

Outdoor Activities: Spending time outside with bare feet on natural surfaces like grass, sand, or dirt is one of the simplest and most direct grounding methods.

Grounding Equipment: If you have limited access to outdoor spaces, grounding devices such as mats, sheets, or patches can be used. These devices use conductive materials to simulate the same electrical contact with the Earth.

Mindful Activities in Nature: Combine grounding with activities such as yoga, meditation, or breathing exercises in an outdoor setting. This combination can enhance both the grounding effect and the mindfulness practice, deepening the mind-body connection.

Nature Immersion: Simply spending time in nature, such as going for a hike, swimming in a lake, or gardening, can also provide grounding effects. Nature immersion has been shown to have numerous health benefits, including stress reduction and improved mood.

Conclusion

In essence, grounding is an accessible and effective way to enhance the mind-body connection. The practice's inherent benefits, including increased mindfulness, stress reduction, improved physical health, and emotional regulation, all contribute to a more robust mind-body dialogue. By incorporating grounding practices into our daily routine, we can better understand and respond to our body's needs, enhancing our overall well-being. As we foster this deeper mind-body connection, we become more in tune with ourselves, facilitating health, balance, and harmony. Grounding ultimately empowers us to take proactive steps towards our holistic health, enriching our lives in the process.

69. GROUNDING AND THE POWER OF INTENTION

Exploring how intention-setting can enhance the Grounding experience and promote manifestation.

Grounding and intention-setting are powerful tools that can be used to create a healthier, more balanced, and fulfilling life. Both practices involve a heightened sense of awareness and connection—grounding with the Earth and our bodies, and intention-setting with our inner desires and goals. This article aims to explore how these two practices can be combined to enhance our grounding experience and harness the power of manifestation.

Understanding Grounding and Intention-Setting

Grounding, or earthing, involves establishing a direct physical connection with the Earth, which can balance our physical and emotional state by stabilizing the electrical environment of our bodies. Intention-setting, on the other hand, is a mindful practice that involves defining and focusing on our desired outcomes or state of being. Intention-setting is a critical step in the process of manifestation—the act of bringing something tangible into your life through belief and expectation.

Grounding as a Foundation for Intention-Setting

Grounding can serve as a fundamental basis for intention-setting, here's how.

Presence: Grounding encourages us to be present in the moment, an essential state for setting clear, focused intentions. When grounded, we are better able to concentrate our thoughts on our desired outcomes without distraction.

Clarity: Grounding can clear our minds, helping us achieve a state of calm and tranquility. This clarity allows us to better identify our true desires and set meaningful, authentic intentions.

Alignment: By connecting us to the Earth and our physical bodies, grounding can help align our physical and emotional states. This alignment fosters coherence between our thoughts, feelings, and actions, which is crucial for effective intention-setting and manifestation.

Energy: The Earth's energy can help revitalize our bodies and minds, boosting our mood and increasing our vibrational frequency. A higher vibration can amplify our intentions and attract positive experiences into our lives.

Integrating Intention-Setting into Grounding Practices

How do we incorporate intention-setting into our grounding practices? Here are some suggestions.

Mindful Meditation: While grounded, practice mindful meditation and set your intentions. Visualize your desires as if they have already materialized. Feel the emotions associated with achieving your desires.

Affirmations: Develop affirmations that reflect your intentions. Recite these affirmations during your grounding session to reinforce your intention and create a powerful emotional connection.

Physical Movements: Combine grounding with physical movements such as yoga or Tai Chi. Before each session, set an intention related to your physical well-being, mindfulness, or emotional balance.

Journaling: While grounding, write down your intentions in a journal. Writing not only helps clarify your intentions but also provides a tangible record that you can reflect on over time.

The Power of Combined Practices

By integrating grounding with intention-setting, we harness the power of both practices. Grounding provides the clarity, presence, alignment, and energy necessary for effective intention-setting. Intention-setting, in turn, directs this grounded energy towards our desired outcomes, amplifying our manifestation efforts.

In essence, grounding can enhance our connection with ourselves and the world around us, while intention-setting can guide us towards our personal growth and achievement goals. When used together, these practices can support our physical and emotional well-being, help us manifest our desires, and empower us to lead more fulfilling lives.

The integration of grounding and intention-setting underscores a vital concept: we have the innate power to shape our lives. By staying grounded and setting clear intentions, we can transform our inner thoughts and desires into our outer reality, cultivating a life that resonates with our deepest values and aspirations.

70. GROUNDING AND THE POWER OF AFFECTION

Discussing the Benefits of Physical Touch and Affection in Conjunction with Grounding Practices

Grounding and affection—two practices that can fundamentally shape and enhance our physical, mental, and emotional well-being. Grounding roots us to the Earth, balancing our energy and reducing stress, while affection, particularly in the form of physical touch, can provide emotional comfort and strengthen interpersonal relationships. Combining these practices can heighten their individual benefits, leading to a more balanced, connected, and emotionally fulfilling life.

Affection, particularly physical touch, is a fundamental human need and a powerful form of communication. It can communicate love, comfort, and support, and its benefits are extensive. Physical affection can trigger the release of oxytocin, the "love hormone," which reduces stress, promotes bonding, and contributes to overall well-being.

The Intersection of Grounding and Affection

Grounding and affection intertwine beautifully in multiple ways, and their integration can be quite impactful:

Stress Reduction: Both grounding and physical affection are known to lower stress. They can reduce cortisol levels, calm the nervous system, and encourage a state of relaxation. Combining these practices can amplify these stress-reducing effects.

Presence: Grounding and affectionate touch both promote presence and mindfulness. They help us focus on the here and now, leading to heightened awareness and appreciation of our surroundings and interactions.

Connection: Grounding connects us with the Earth, while affection connects us with others. Together, they foster a sense of oneness and interconnection, nurturing our relationship with ourselves, others, and nature.

Integrating Affection into Grounding Practices

Incorporating affectionate touch into grounding practices can be a beautiful experience. Here are a few ways to do so.

Grounding with a Loved One: Practicing grounding with a partner, family member, or friend can enhance the experience. Holding hands or hugging while grounded can deepen your emotional connection while sharing the grounding benefits.

Touching the Earth: When grounding, try to engage with the Earth more affectionately. Feel the grass, sand, or soil under your hands and feet. Acknowledge the connection and appreciate the nourishment that Earth provides.

Pet Therapy: Pets can provide affection and comfort. Grounding with your pet can be a joyful experience, fostering a deeper bond with your animal companion while you both enjoy the grounding benefits.

Grounding Massage: Incorporating a grounding massage into your routine can be beneficial. Use grounding oils while massaging to amplify the benefits of both grounding and affectionate touch.

The Synergistic Power of Grounding and Affection

The synergy of grounding and affection offers powerful benefits for our well-being. The physiological benefits include decreased inflammation, improved immune response, and stress reduction. Simultaneously, the emotional benefits include increased feelings of love, connection, empathy, and understanding.

Furthermore, practicing grounding and affection simultaneously can also enhance our relationships. Shared experiences of grounding can foster deeper connections with loved ones, while the expression of physical affection during these practices can create a nurturing and supportive environment.

In conclusion, grounding and affection are two powerful practices that, when combined, can offer significant benefits. By incorporating affectionate touch into our grounding routines, we can enhance our physical and emotional health, foster deeper connections with others, and cultivate a more profound appreciation for the natural world. As we explore this integrative practice, we open ourselves to a deeper level of healing and connection, embodying the essence of what it means to be human in harmony with the Earth.

71. GROUNDING AND THE POWER OF SELF-CARE

Investigating How Grounding Practices Can Be Incorporated Into Self-Care Routines for Enhanced Well-being

In an increasingly chaotic and fast-paced world, self-care has become a crucial component of maintaining our physical, emotional, and mental health. One effective practice that is rapidly gaining recognition for its ability to improve well-being is grounding. This essay explores the importance of grounding and its incorporation into self-care routines for enhanced well-being.

Grounding has been shown to have numerous benefits, including reduced stress levels, improved sleep quality, decreased inflammation, and enhanced immune function. The core concept behind these benefits is the neutralization of harmful free radicals and the balancing of the body's bioelectrical environment.

Grounding and Self-Care

Self-care, in its simplest form, is the conscious act of taking care of our well-being and happiness, in particular during periods of stress. It involves various practices aimed at promoting physical, emotional, and mental health. Grounding can be a vital addition to a self-care regimen due to its substantial benefits.

Integrating grounding into a self-care routine could look like this:

Morning Grounding: Starting the day with grounding can set a calm and focused tone for the day ahead. This could involve a barefoot walk in the garden, sitting under a tree, or even gardening.

Grounding During Exercise: Engaging in grounding exercises, such as yoga or Tai Chi, outdoors enhances the benefits of the exercise and provides grounding simultaneously.

Evening Grounding: Grounding before bed can improve sleep quality. This could be achieved by standing barefoot outside and taking several deep breaths, ideally looking at the setting sun.

Grounding Breaks: Taking grounding breaks during a stressful day can provide relief and reduce anxiety levels.

Benefits of Incorporating Grounding into Self-Care

Incorporating grounding into self-care routines offers several benefits.

Enhanced Physical Health: Grounding has been linked to various physical health benefits, such as improved sleep, reduced inflammation, and enhanced wound healing.

Mental and Emotional Well-being: Grounding can lower stress levels, reduce anxiety, and improve mood, contributing to better mental and emotional health.

Increased Mindfulness: Grounding encourages mindfulness by requiring us to focus on the present moment, our connection with the Earth, and the sensations within our bodies.

Promotion of Balance: Grounding promotes balance in our lives by encouraging us to spend more time in nature, away from the distractions and stresses of modern life.

Boosts Immunity: Grounding improves immune function, thus helping to fend off illnesses and maintain overall health.

Grounding and the Future of Self-Care

As our understanding of health evolves, it becomes increasingly clear that our connection to nature plays a significant role in our well-being. Grounding offers a powerful yet simple method of enhancing this connection and integrating it into our self-care routines. It requires no special equipment or substantial time commitment, making it an accessible practice for many.

Self-care is an investment in our well-being, and grounding is a significant asset in that investment. It extends beyond merely taking care of ourselves, fostering a deeper connection with the Earth and promoting a greater sense of balance and harmony in our lives.

In conclusion, grounding is a powerful practice with significant potential for enhancing our well-being when incorporated into self-care routines. Whether it's spending time barefoot in the grass, swimming in a natural body of water, or grounding during exercise, the simple act of connecting with the Earth can provide substantial health benefits and contribute to a greater sense of peace and contentment in our lives.

72. GROUNDING AND THE POWER OF SELF-COMPASSION

Discussing How Grounding Practices Can Support Self-Compassion and Self-Love

In a world fraught with stress, pressure, and an incessant demand for perfection, we often forget to extend kindness and compassion towards ourselves. However, self-compassion and self-love are fundamental to our well-being and mental health. One practice that can cultivate these elements is grounding. This essay delves into the subject of how grounding practices can nurture self-compassion and self-love.

Proponents of grounding assert that it promotes numerous health benefits, such as improved sleep, reduced inflammation, decreased stress, and better mood regulation. Moreover, grounding provides an opportunity for introspection and presence in the moment, further contributing to mental health and emotional well-being.

Grounding and Self-Compassion

Self-compassion is the ability to extend understanding, acceptance, and kindness towards oneself, especially during periods of failure or perceived inadequacy. Grounding can play a pivotal role in nurturing self-compassion in several ways:

Promoting Mindfulness: Grounding requires presence in the moment, which is a cornerstone of mindfulness. Through grounding, we become more aware of our thoughts, emotions, and bodily sensations without judgment, fostering self-compassion.

Connecting with Nature: Grounding helps us connect with nature, which can provide a soothing effect and promote feelings of well-being. This connection can remind us that just like nature, we too have cycles of growth, stagnation, decay, and renewal, fostering a compassionate acceptance of our human nature.

Reducing Stress and Anxiety: Grounding has been linked to reduced stress and anxiety levels. When we are less stressed, we are better able to show compassion towards ourselves.

Cultivating Self-Kindness: Grounding allows us time to pause, step back, and engage in self-care, thereby fostering self-kindness. This practice reinforces that we are worthy of care and compassion.

Benefits of Grounding for Self-Compassion and Self-Love

Incorporating grounding into our routine can bring about numerous benefits.

Mental Health: Grounding can improve mood, reduce anxiety, and manage depression, contributing to better mental health and improved self-perception.

Physical Health: The potential physical benefits of grounding, including improved sleep and reduced inflammation, can enhance our physical well-being, fostering a better relationship with our bodies.

Emotional Resilience: Grounding can support emotional resilience by helping us stay centered during times of stress, thereby enabling us to navigate difficult emotions with more compassion and understanding.

Enhanced Self-Worth: Grounding, by promoting self-care and connection with the earth, can enhance feelings of self-worth and self-love.

The Intersection of Grounding, Self-Compassion, and Self-Love

Grounding, self-compassion, and self-love intersect at the point of our fundamental humanity. As we connect with the earth, we are reminded that we are part of the natural world, subject to the same laws of growth and change. This understanding fosters a compassionate view of our shortcomings and challenges, affirming that they are part of the shared human experience.

Through grounding, we can learn to extend the same understanding and compassion to ourselves that we naturally extend to the earth and other living things. We can embrace our imperfections, celebrate our uniqueness, and nurture a profound sense of self-love.

In conclusion, grounding is a powerful practice that supports the cultivation of self-compassion and self-love. As we connect with the earth and ground ourselves in the present moment, we are afforded an opportunity to extend kindness, understanding, and love towards ourselves. In doing so, we not only enhance our physical and mental health but also nurture a compassionate relationship with ourselves that is central to overall well-being. Grounding is a practice of not just reconnection with the earth, but a reconnection with ourselves in the most compassionate and loving way.

73. GROUNDING AND THE POWER OF FORGIVENESS

Grounding and the Power of Forgiveness: Exploring How Grounding Practices Can Support the Process of Forgiveness and Emotional Healing

In the journey of life, hurt and betrayal are often inevitable. These painful experiences can lead to lingering resentment, anger, and emotional distress. The process of forgiveness is a powerful means to healing these emotional wounds and regaining inner peace. Grounding, a therapeutic practice that connects us physically and psychologically to the earth, can greatly support this process. This exploration will delve into how grounding can aid the process of forgiveness and emotional healing.

Understanding Grounding

Grounding, also known as earthing, involves direct contact with the earth's surface. This practice harnesses the earth's natural electric charge to promote physiological and psychological well-being. Walking barefoot on grass, swimming in a natural body of water, or simply sitting or lying on the earth can facilitate grounding. Research suggests that grounding can provide numerous health benefits, including stress reduction, improved sleep, reduced inflammation, and enhanced mood regulation. Beyond the physical, grounding also promotes mental tranquility and emotional stability, key factors in facilitating forgiveness.

Grounding and Forgiveness

Forgiveness, an intentional process of letting go of resentment and thoughts of revenge, requires a high level of emotional maturity and self-awareness. It is not about condoning or forgetting the hurt inflicted, but rather about freeing oneself from the damaging hold of bitterness. Here's how grounding can support this process:

Promoting Mindfulness: Grounding naturally fosters mindfulness, a state of active, open attention to the present. This mindfulness can allow us to observe our feelings of hurt and resentment without judgment, opening the door to forgiveness.

Reducing Stress and Anxiety: Grounding has been shown to reduce stress and anxiety. Lower stress levels can promote emotional balance, making the process of forgiveness more accessible.

Cultivating Empathy: By fostering a connection with nature and the larger universe, grounding can help cultivate empathy, a critical element in the process of forgiveness.

Enhancing Emotional Resilience: Grounding can enhance emotional resilience, equipping us with the strength to face our pain, forgive, and move forward.

Benefits of Grounding for Forgiveness and Emotional Healing

The benefits of grounding in facilitating forgiveness and emotional healing are multifaceted:

Emotional Freedom: By supporting the process of forgiveness, grounding can help us let go of destructive emotions like resentment and bitterness, leading to emotional freedom.

Improved Relationships: Forgiveness often results in improved relationships. As grounding supports forgiveness, it indirectly contributes to healthier, more fulfilling relationships.

Greater Peace of Mind: Holding onto resentment often robs us of peace of mind. Through facilitating forgiveness, grounding can help restore this peace.

Enhanced Well-Being: By supporting emotional healing and reducing stress, grounding contributes to overall physical and psychological well-being.

Grounding, Forgiveness, and Emotional Healing: The Intersection

Grounding, forgiveness, and emotional healing intersect in the quest for inner peace and well-being. As we connect with the earth through grounding, we tap into a natural source of tranquility and stability. This can help us face our hurt and resentment, paving the way for forgiveness and subsequent emotional healing. Through this process, we not only let go of destructive emotions but also reclaim our inner peace and emotional freedom.

In conclusion, grounding is a potent practice that supports forgiveness and emotional healing. It fosters mindfulness, reduces stress and anxiety, cultivates empathy, and enhances emotional resilience, all of which contributes to the process of forgiveness. Through grounding, we can better navigate the often-complex journey of forgiveness, leading to profound emotional healing, peace of mind, and overall well-being. Thus, grounding serves as a pathway not only to the earth but also to forgiveness and emotional liberation.

74. GROUNDING AND THE POWER OF GRATITUDE

Discussing the Benefits of Practicing Gratitude in Conjunction with Grounding Practices

The practices of grounding and gratitude, while seemingly separate, are deeply interconnected and can greatly complement one another. Grounding, the process of connecting with the earth's natural energy, brings numerous health benefits, including stress reduction, mood stabilization, and improved sleep. Simultaneously, gratitude, an emotional response to positivity in one's life, contributes to improved mental well-being and satisfaction. By practicing gratitude in conjunction with grounding, individuals can experience a heightened state of wellness and contentment.

Gratitude and Its Power

Gratitude, as a practice, involves regularly acknowledging and appreciating the positive aspects of life. This could be as significant as appreciating one's good health or as subtle as being grateful for a sunny day. Studies suggest that regular gratitude practices can enhance mental health, boost happiness, decrease depression, and even improve quality of sleep. Furthermore, gratitude can facilitate the nurturing of relationships, lead to increased empathy, and foster resilience.

Integrating Grounding and Gratitude

The fusion of grounding and gratitude can lead to a heightened state of wellness. Grounding provides a platform for individuals to slow down, immerse in the present, and reconnect with the environment. It serves as an anchor, stabilizing emotions and providing a sense of calm. This serene state, established through grounding, forms a conducive environment to engage in gratitude practices. As individuals ground themselves, they can leverage this tranquility to reflect on the positive aspects of their lives, fostering a deep sense of gratitude.

Benefits of Grounding and Gratitude Practices

The combined benefits of grounding and gratitude practices are profound.

Enhanced Emotional Well-being: Both grounding and gratitude practices contribute to emotional well-being. Grounding helps to reduce negative emotions, such as anxiety and stress, while gratitude encourages a positive outlook.

Improved Physical Health: Grounding has been linked to various physical health benefits, including improved sleep and reduced inflammation. Simultaneously, gratitude can lead to better self-care practices, further contributing to physical health.

Greater Life Satisfaction: Gratitude helps to foster a positive attitude and appreciation for life. When combined with the calming effects of grounding, individuals can experience heightened life satisfaction.

Increased Connection: Both practices promote a deeper connection - grounding with the earth and environment, and gratitude with oneself and others.

Boosted Resilience: Grounding and gratitude can foster resilience, enhancing one's ability to navigate through life's challenges.

Grounding, Gratitude, and Wellness: A Symbiotic Relationship

Grounding and gratitude form a symbiotic relationship that can greatly enhance overall wellness. Grounding offers a calming platform conducive to reflection and the practice of gratitude. In turn, gratitude can heighten the benefits derived from grounding by fostering positivity and satisfaction. This mutual enhancement amplifies the impacts of both practices, contributing to increased physical and emotional well-being, heightened life satisfaction, and boosted resilience.

In conclusion, grounding and gratitude are powerful practices individually. However, when combined, they create a synergy that multiplies their benefits, providing a potent tool for enhancing wellness. By integrating gratitude practices into grounding routines, individuals can nurture positivity, improve health, and cultivate an overall sense of contentment and connection with the world around them. Ultimately, the harmonious union of grounding and gratitude provides a path towards balanced, joyful, and meaningful living.

75. GROUNDING AND THE POWER OF CONNECTION

Investigating how Grounding Practices can Foster a Deeper Sense of Connection with Oneself, Others, and the Environment

Our modern world, marked by technological advancements and a fast-paced lifestyle, often makes us feel disconnected. Disconnected from ourselves, from others, and significantly, from nature. Grounding practices, however, present an antidote to this sense of disconnection, fostering a deeper bond with our inner selves, others around us, and the world we inhabit.

The Three Connections

The power of grounding lies in its capacity to facilitate three critical connections – with ourselves, others, and the environment. Each connection forms a part of a holistic approach to wellness, with grounding serving as a common thread weaving them together.

Self-Connection

One of the primary benefits of grounding is its capacity to deepen our connection with ourselves. Through grounding, we engage with the present moment, distancing ourselves from distractions and stressors. This encourages mindfulness and introspection, allowing us to become more in tune with our thoughts, emotions, and physical sensations. The result is enhanced self-awareness and understanding, serving as a foundation for personal growth and self-improvement.

Interpersonal Connection

Grounding also holds the potential to strengthen our relationships with others. As grounding practices cultivate mindfulness, empathy, and compassion, they inherently promote healthier, more meaningful interpersonal interactions. When we are grounded, we are better able to listen, understand, and respond to others, fostering deeper connections and enriching our social lives.

Environmental Connection

Perhaps the most intuitive connection fostered through grounding is the one with our environment. As we physically connect with the Earth and immerse ourselves in nature during grounding practices, we develop a heightened appreciation for the natural world. This environmental connection can lead to increased environmental consciousness, prompting actions and choices that respect and preserve our shared planet.

The Synergy of Connections

These three connections—self, others, and environment—do not exist in isolation. Instead, they interact synergistically to promote holistic wellbeing. Grounding serves as a catalyst for this synergy, fostering each connection and enabling them to collectively contribute to a more fulfilling and balanced life.

Grounding for Enhanced Connection

To harness the power of grounding for enhanced connection, regular practice is key. Choose grounding activities that resonate with you—be it forest bathing, barefoot walking, or gardening—

and incorporate them into your daily routine. Remember, the goal is to physically connect with the Earth while fostering mindfulness and presence.

Conclusion

In our increasingly fragmented and fast-paced world, grounding offers a powerful means to foster a deeper sense of connection — with ourselves, others, and the environment. Through grounding practices, we can enhance self-awareness, enrich interpersonal relationships, and cultivate environmental consciousness. By embracing the power of grounding, we can navigate towards a more connected, mindful, and fulfilling existence. The journey of grounding, therefore, is not merely a path towards better health but a voyage of reconnection, bringing us back to our roots, enhancing our understanding of ourselves and the world around us, and restoring the essential bonds that nourish our lives.

76. GROUNDING AND THE POWER OF EMPATHY

Discussing how Grounding practices can enhance empathy and compassion for others.

In a world that often seems polarized and fragmented, the power of empathy and compassion feels more crucial than ever. Grounding practices, or earthing, can serve as a vehicle for cultivating these traits, enabling individuals to feel a deeper connection and understanding of the emotions and experiences of others. This article explores how the practice of grounding can enhance empathy and compassion, making it an integral part of our emotional intelligence and human connectedness.

Empathy and Grounding

Empathy, the ability to understand and share the feelings of others, is a trait that grounding can nurture in several ways. The act of grounding brings about a greater sense of mindfulness and presence, both of which are fundamental to empathy. Mindfulness allows us to be fully engaged in the present moment and to be more aware of our thoughts, emotions, and senses. This heightened awareness makes it easier to recognize and understand the feelings and experiences of others.

By practicing grounding, individuals cultivate a habit of introspection and self-reflection, enabling them to better recognize their emotions and understand how their actions affect others. This improved emotional awareness can enhance empathetic responses, as individuals are better equipped to 'step into the shoes' of others, feeling their joy, pain, excitement, or despair.

Compassion and Grounding

While empathy refers to the understanding and sharing of feelings, compassion involves the willingness to relieve the suffering of others. Grounding can enhance compassion in a similar manner to empathy. The practice encourages individuals to develop a sense of oneness with the world around them, including their fellow beings. This feeling of interconnectedness fosters a natural inclination to alleviate others' pain and suffering, leading to greater compassion.

Moreover, grounding's emphasis on connection with nature can contribute to the cultivation of compassion. The beauty and tranquility of nature often evoke feelings of peace, love, and kindness, emotions that are conducive to compassionate behavior. When grounded, people tend to be more receptive to these feelings, using them to fuel acts of kindness and consideration towards others.

Practical Tips for Enhancing Empathy and Compassion Through Grounding

To utilize grounding as a means to enhance empathy and compassion, there are a few practices one can adopt:

Nature Meditations: This involves meditating in a natural environment, focusing on the sounds, smells, and sensations around you. This practice cultivates mindfulness, a key component of empathy and compassion.

Walking Barefoot: Walking barefoot on the Earth allows you to absorb its natural energies, fostering a sense of connectedness and empathy with all life forms.

Practicing Mindful Observance: Observing nature mindfully, watching the trees, the sky, or any aspect of the natural world, can enhance feelings of interconnectedness and empathy.

Journaling: Writing about your grounding experiences, emotions, and reflections can help to process feelings and enhance your understanding of yourself and others.

Conclusion

Empathy and compassion are two fundamental traits that make our world a better, more connected place. Grounding, with its inherent capacity to foster mindfulness, interconnectedness, and emotional awareness, provides a unique avenue for enhancing these traits. As we embrace grounding practices, we not only reap individual physical and mental health benefits but also contribute to a more empathetic and compassionate world. The power of grounding thus extends beyond the individual, strengthening our bonds with others and making the world a more understanding, kind, and supportive place for all.

77. GROUNDING AND THE POWER OF BOUNDARIES

Exploring how Grounding practices can support the development of healthy boundaries and self-care.

Life in the 21st century, marked by relentless schedules, constant connectivity, and a myriad of expectations, can often leave individuals feeling overwhelmed and out of touch with their needs and desires. Setting healthy boundaries, therefore, has emerged as a critical aspect of personal well-being and self-care. This piece examines how grounding practices can support the development of these essential boundaries, fostering emotional stability and overall health.

The Power of Boundaries

Personal boundaries act as guidelines, rules, or limits that an individual creates to identify safe and permissible ways for others to behave towards them. They also determine how one will respond when these limits are violated. Boundaries might concern emotions, energy, time, or personal space, and they vary from person to person. They are key to maintaining a balanced life, as they help protect one's mental, emotional, and physical health.

Grounding and Boundaries

Grounding can be an invaluable tool in setting and maintaining boundaries. By promoting mindfulness and body awareness, grounding can help individuals understand their needs better, which is the first step in setting healthy boundaries. Furthermore, the serenity experienced during grounding can provide the mental space to assess current boundaries and the effects they have on one's life.

Practical Ways Grounding Supports Boundary Setting

Mindfulness and Self-Awareness: Grounding naturally encourages mindfulness and presence, which enables an individual to recognize their feelings, needs, and limits. Understanding these is the first step to establishing healthy boundaries.

Boosting Self-Esteem and Assertiveness: Grounding practices can help individuals boost their self-esteem and assertiveness, essential traits for enforcing boundaries. Feeling grounded and connected with nature can foster a sense of self-worth, empowering individuals to defend their boundaries.

Reducing Stress and Anxiety: Grounding can help alleviate stress and anxiety, which often interfere with the ability to maintain boundaries. When one's mind is relaxed and focused, they are better equipped to communicate their boundaries effectively.

Developing Emotional Resilience: Regular grounding practices can enhance emotional resilience, helping individuals cope when their boundaries are tested or violated.

Implementing Grounding in Boundary Setting and Self-Care

Practicing grounding with the intention of supporting boundary setting involves being mindful of one's emotional and mental states and needs during the practice. Here are some steps that can be helpful:

Begin with Awareness: As you engage in grounding, pay attention to your feelings and emotions. Are you feeling exhausted, stressed, or perhaps overwhelmed? These emotions could signal a need for better boundaries.

Reflect on Your Boundaries: Use the calm and clarity provided by grounding to reflect on your current boundaries. Are they serving your needs? Where do you need to establish new boundaries or reinforce existing ones?

Practice Assertiveness: Grounding can serve as a rehearsal space for assertiveness. In your grounded state, visualize yourself communicating your boundaries confidently and calmly.

Take Regular Grounding Breaks: Make grounding a regular part of your routine. Just as you might take regular breaks to rest or eat, schedule grounding breaks to check in with yourself and your boundaries.

Conclusion

Developing and maintaining healthy boundaries is crucial for personal well-being and effective self-care. Grounding practices, by promoting mindfulness, self-esteem, and emotional resilience, can offer significant support in this aspect. As individuals embrace the grounding lifestyle, they not only enjoy improved physical health but also empower themselves to cultivate a balanced life with respectful and beneficial boundaries. Ultimately, grounding practices hold the potential to enhance not only our connection with the Earth but also with our true selves and our needs.

78. GROUNDING AND THE POWER OF CREATIVITY

Investigating How Grounding Practices Can Enhance Creativity and Artistic Expression.

In a world where innovation is a central driver of both personal and professional growth, creativity is a highly sought-after asset. Yet, with myriad responsibilities and distractions, finding ways to tap into and nurture our creative capacities can prove challenging. This exploration focuses on how grounding practices can foster creativity and boost artistic expression, unlocking a new dimension of human potential.

An Overview of Grounding

At its core, grounding (or earthing) is the process of physically connecting with the Earth to draw from its natural energy. This connection is usually achieved by walking barefoot on the Earth's surface, gardening, or any other activity that puts you in direct contact with the ground. Grounding has been linked to various health benefits, including reduced inflammation, stress relief, and improved sleep. However, its capacity to stimulate creativity remains an underexplored area of interest.

Creativity and Its Importance

Creativity is the ability to produce original and valuable ideas or solutions. It's not confined to artistic or musical expression; creativity encompasses problem-solving, innovative thinking, and the ability to envision new possibilities across all fields of human endeavor. By enhancing creativity, individuals can enrich their personal lives, contribute more effectively to their workplaces, and navigate life's challenges with greater ease and success.

How Grounding Enhances Creativity

Grounding practices can stimulate creativity in several ways:

Promoting Mindfulness: Grounding inherently promotes mindfulness, the practice of being fully present and engaged with the current moment. This state of mind opens the door to new perceptions and ideas, encouraging creative thinking.

Reducing Stress and Anxiety: Creativity often struggles to flourish in high-stress environments. Grounding has been shown to reduce stress and anxiety, creating a mental landscape where creative thoughts can take root and grow.

Improving Sleep Quality: As grounding enhances sleep quality, it allows the brain to rest and rejuvenate, leading to heightened cognitive functioning and creative thinking the following day.

Strengthening Connection with Nature: Grounding fosters a deeper connection with nature, which has been linked to increased creativity. The natural world often inspires new ideas and perspectives, feeding the creative process.

Practical Steps to Leverage Grounding for Creativity

To capitalize on the creative benefits of grounding, consider the following tips:

Regular Grounding Sessions: Incorporate grounding into your daily routine. This could involve walking barefoot in your backyard, spending time in a garden, or taking a break in a nearby park.

Mindful Observation: During your grounding session, try to observe your surroundings mindfully. Notice the colors, sounds, and textures around you. These sensory experiences can inspire new ideas and creative perspectives.

Combine Grounding with Creative Activities: Try combining grounding with creative activities such as sketching, writing, or brainstorming ideas. The relaxed mental state induced by grounding can enhance these activities.

Use Grounding as a Pre-Creative Ritual: Utilize grounding as a ritual before diving into creative work. This practice can help clear your mind and stimulate a creative mindset.

Conclusion

In the quest for creativity, grounding emerges as a compelling ally. By reducing stress, fostering mindfulness, and enhancing our connection with nature, grounding can help unlock our inherent creative abilities. Through regular practice, individuals may not only experience improved health and wellbeing but also witness a marked enhancement in their creative output and artistic expression. Therefore, grounding deserves recognition as a natural, accessible, and effective means of nurturing creativity in our increasingly complex world.

79. GROUNDING AND THE POWER OF MOVEMENT

Discussing the Benefits of Incorporating Movement and Physical Activity into Grounding Practices

In the realm of holistic health and wellness, grounding and physical activity each have an important role to play. Grounding, the practice of physically connecting with the Earth, and movement, a key component of overall health, are two practices that, when integrated, can yield potent benefits. This exploration delves into the intersection of grounding and movement, shedding light on the multifaceted benefits of incorporating physical activity into grounding practices.

The Role of Movement in Health

Movement, a broad term encompassing various forms of physical activity, is vital to our health. Regular movement improves cardiovascular health, boosts mental wellness, supports weight management, and enhances overall quality of life. Whether it's rigorous exercise or low-intensity activities like walking or stretching, any form of movement contributes to a healthier, more balanced lifestyle.

The Intersection of Grounding and Movement

The synergy of grounding and movement presents a unique approach to health and wellness. By incorporating physical activity into grounding practices, we can potentially enhance the benefits of both, resulting in improved physical health, emotional balance, and cognitive function.

Here's how the combination works

Enhanced Health Benefits: The physical activity involved in grounding exercises — like barefoot walking or yoga on the grass — combines the benefits of grounding with those of exercise. This may result in improved cardiovascular health, increased strength and flexibility, and better balance and coordination.

Reduced Inflammation: Grounding has been linked to decreased inflammation. Combined with the anti-inflammatory effects of exercise, grounding movement practices can offer a powerful approach to managing inflammation-related conditions.

Stress Relief: Movement is known to boost mood and alleviate stress by promoting the release of endorphins, our body's natural mood elevators. Coupled with the stress-reducing effects of grounding, physical activities performed while grounded can contribute to enhanced emotional well-being.

Cognitive Benefits: Regular physical activity promotes better brain health, enhancing cognitive functions like memory and attention. When combined with grounding, which has also been associated with improved mental clarity, movement practices can offer a potent cognitive boost.

Incorporating Movement into Grounding Practices

There are numerous ways to incorporate movement into your grounding practices.

Barefoot Walking or Running: Walking or running barefoot on grass, sand, or soil not only grounds you but also engages your muscles, offering cardiovascular benefits.

Grounding Yoga or Stretching: Performing yoga poses or stretching exercises outdoors on the ground can combine the physical benefits of these activities with the therapeutic effects of grounding.

Outdoor Workouts: Consider doing your usual workout routine outdoors, barefoot if possible. Whether it's calisthenics, high-intensity interval training (HIIT), or resistance training, doing so on a natural surface can integrate grounding's benefits.

Nature Hikes: Hiking barefoot or with minimalist footwear allows for grounding while offering the physical benefits of this exercise. It also provides opportunities for mindfulness and connection with nature.

Conclusion

The integration of grounding and movement presents a compelling blend for health and well-being. This harmonious pairing enhances the physical, emotional, and cognitive benefits attributed to each practice individually, promoting an enriched sense of wellness. As such, incorporating movement into grounding practices offers a dynamic, holistic approach to nurturing our health—providing yet another compelling reason to kick off our shoes and engage with the natural world.

80. GROUNDING AND THE POWER OF NUTRITION

Exploring How Grounding Practices Can Be Complemented by a Healthy and Nourishing Diet.

In the pursuit of holistic wellness, the intricate intertwining of various practices is often highlighted, including grounding and nutrition. Grounding, the practice of physically connecting oneself with the Earth, has been recognized for its numerous health benefits. Similarly, nutrition plays an integral role in maintaining physical health and emotional well-being. Exploring the synergistic potential of these practices provides a comprehensive approach towards holistic health. Here, we delve into how grounding can be complemented and potentially amplified by a healthy and nourishing diet.

The Role of Nutrition in Health

Nutrition is an undisputed cornerstone of health. What we eat significantly affects our physical health, influencing weight, energy levels, and the risk of many diseases. Furthermore, it impacts our mental and emotional well-being. A balanced, nutrient-rich diet can help manage mood, improve cognitive function, and contribute to overall quality of life.

Grounding and Nutrition: A Synergistic Approach

The integration of grounding and nutritional practices presents an exciting avenue for promoting health and wellness. Here's how these two concepts intertwine.

Amplified Health Benefits: Grounding is believed to promote better sleep, reduce inflammation, and help manage stress. Nutrition also plays a crucial role in these areas. A balanced diet strengthens the immune system, supports mental health, and provides the energy needed for the body to function optimally. Thus, the practices of grounding and maintaining a healthy diet can amplify each other's health benefits.

Antioxidant Effects: Grounding is thought to provide antioxidant effects by neutralizing free radicals. Antioxidants are also abundant in a healthy diet, particularly in fruits, vegetables, nuts, and seeds. This common characteristic suggests a synergistic potential in coupling grounding practices with a diet rich in antioxidants.

Stress Management: Both grounding and nutrition play roles in stress management. Grounding is suggested to activate the parasympathetic nervous system, inducing relaxation. Simultaneously, certain nutrients, like omega-3 fatty acids and B vitamins, have been linked to stress reduction. This shared attribute makes a combined approach potentially more effective.

Inflammation Reduction: Grounding has been associated with decreased inflammation, as has a nutrient-rich diet. Foods high in omega-3 fatty acids, antioxidants, and other anti-inflammatory compounds can help manage inflammation. Combining grounding with such a diet may offer a potent approach to inflammation reduction.

Implementing Grounding and Nutritional Practices

Incorporating grounding into a healthy lifestyle can be as simple as spending time barefoot in nature. Walk on the grass, swim in the sea, or just sit with your hands touching the Earth.

Complementing this with a healthy diet involves consuming a variety of nutrient-rich foods. Include a rainbow of fruits and vegetables, lean proteins, healthy fats, and whole grains. Pay attention to hydration and consider the timing of meals in relation to your grounding practices.

It might also be beneficial to consume a nutrient-rich meal or snack after a grounding session, similar to refueling after a workout. This can replenish energy stores and provide nutrients needed for recovery and repair.

Conclusion

Grounding and nutrition each have a unique role in promoting health and well-being. Yet, their potential combined impact suggests a synergistic effect that can further enhance health benefits. This holistic approach highlights the power of integrating various wellness practices. By understanding and implementing grounding and nutritional practices together, we take a comprehensive, multi-faceted approach to health and wellness — one that respects the interconnected nature of our bodies and our environment.

81. GROUNDING AND THE POWER OF MINDFUL EATING

Investigating How Mindful Eating Practices Can Enhance the Grounding Experience and Promote Overall Health

The realms of holistic wellness and mindfulness have expanded to various aspects of life, one being our dietary habits. Grounding or earthing, a practice of reconnecting ourselves with the Earth's energy, is known to have several benefits, including reducing inflammation, enhancing sleep, and reducing stress. Similarly, mindful eating, which emphasizes being fully present during meals, encourages healthier eating habits and an improved relationship with food. This exploration dives into the symbiotic relationship between grounding and mindful eating, showing how the latter can enhance the grounding experience and promote overall health.

The Practice of Mindful Eating

Mindful eating is a practice that involves being fully present during meals, tuning into the sensory experiences of eating, and listening to the body's hunger and fullness cues. By slowing down and savoring each bite, mindful eating can help individuals develop a healthier relationship with food, reduce overeating, enhance digestion, and increase enjoyment of food.

How Mindful Eating Complements Grounding

The combination of grounding and mindful eating can enhance the overall grounding experience and further contribute to holistic health. Here's how these two practices align.

Presence and Awareness: Both grounding and mindful eating cultivate a deeper sense of presence and awareness. While grounding connects us to the Earth and our physical environment, mindful eating brings us back to ourselves and our internal experiences. Together, these practices can foster an amplified state of mindfulness, strengthening the connection between our bodies and our environment.

Stress Reduction: Both practices are recognized for their stress-reducing qualities. Grounding is believed to have calming effects by shifting the body towards the parasympathetic nervous system, the system responsible for rest and digestion. Simultaneously, mindful eating can reduce stress by transforming eating into a more relaxed, enjoyable experience. The combination of these practices can create a powerful tool for stress management.

Improved Digestion: Grounding, through its connection to the parasympathetic nervous system, can support improved digestion. Mindful eating also supports digestion by encouraging slower eating and thorough chewing, allowing the digestive system to work more effectively. Combining these practices may offer a comprehensive approach to improving digestive health.

Integrating Grounding and Mindful Eating into Daily Life

Combining grounding and mindful eating can start with small, daily practices. Begin your day by grounding, perhaps through a barefoot walk outside. Following this, have your meal mindfully, paying attention to each bite, savoring the flavors, and acknowledging the nourishment the food provides your body.

Try to eat outdoors when possible. The natural environment can enhance the grounding experience and make mindful eating easier. The sights, sounds, and smells of nature can enrich the sensory experience of eating.

Make your grounding and mindful eating practices regular habits. Consistency can cultivate a deeper connection with the Earth and your body. As your awareness increases, you may find your food choices changing towards more nourishing and wholesome options, further supporting your overall health.

Conclusion

In today's fast-paced world, practices that promote mindfulness and connection to nature are more crucial than ever. Grounding and mindful eating offer ways to slow down, reconnect with our bodies and the Earth, and enhance our health in a holistic way. These practices remind us of our intrinsic connection with nature and the importance of nurturing our bodies with mindful attention. They represent an integrated approach to health, highlighting the inseparable connection between our bodies and the world in which we live.

82. GROUNDING AND THE POWER OF MINDFUL COMMUNICATION

Discussing how Grounding practices can support mindful communication and enhance relationships.

Mindful communication and grounding are both practices rooted in the philosophy of mindfulness, the awareness of the present moment without judgment. This awareness allows one to engage fully with their experiences, enhancing the quality of their interactions and relationships. By cultivating mindfulness through grounding and applying it to our communication, we can foster meaningful connections with others. This article delves into the intertwined relationship between grounding and mindful communication, and how these practices can mutually enhance each other to better our relationships and interpersonal communication.

Grounding: A Reconnection with Earth

Grounding, or earthing, is a therapeutic technique that involves doing activities that "ground" or electrically reconnect you to the earth. This practice hinges on the theory that our bodies are meant to be in contact with the earth regularly, with direct skin-to-earth contact serving as a conduit for the Earth's electrons. Grounding is believed to have multiple health benefits, including reducing inflammation, increasing energy, and lowering stress and anxiety levels.

Mindful Communication: The Art of Presence in Interactions

Mindful communication, or conscious communication, goes beyond the mere exchange of words. It involves fully being in the moment and actively listening to the other person, conveying your message with clarity, empathy, and respect, and being aware of non-verbal cues. This type of communication fosters understanding, strengthens relationships, and minimizes misunderstandings and conflicts.

Interweaving Grounding and Mindful Communication

The practices of grounding and mindful communication interconnect seamlessly, each enhancing the other to create deeper, more meaningful interactions. Here's how these practices relate:

Enhanced Presence: Grounding allows us to be more present by bringing our focus to our connection with the earth. This heightened sense of presence can carry over into our interactions with others. Through mindful communication, we can maintain this presence, giving our full attention to the person we are communicating with, creating a more meaningful and effective exchange.

Reduced Reactivity: Grounding is known for its calming effect on our nervous system. By reducing anxiety and stress, grounding helps us be less reactive and more responsive, leading to mindful communication. When we are not hijacked by our emotional responses, we can respond more thoughtfully, fostering better understanding and harmony in our relationships.

Enhanced Empathy: By practicing grounding, we become more attuned to our feelings and thoughts. This increased self-awareness can translate into greater empathy for others, an essential aspect of mindful communication. When we understand our own emotions better, we can more easily relate to what others are feeling.

Incorporating Grounding into Mindful Communication Practices

To combine the practices of grounding and mindful communication, you can start by grounding yourself before engaging in any significant conversations or interactions. Spend a few moments outside, barefoot if possible, focusing on your connection with the Earth. This practice can help you enter a calmer, more present state of mind.

During conversations, try to maintain the sense of presence you cultivated through grounding. Fully focus on the other person, paying attention to their words, tone of voice, and body language. Respond thoughtfully rather than reacting impulsively.

Also, consider incorporating grounding practices during conversations, especially during challenging or intense discussions. Taking a few moments to mentally reconnect with the earth can help restore calm and presence.

83. GROUNDING AND THE POWER OF MINDFUL PARENTING

Exploring how Grounding practices can support mindful parenting and enhance family relationships.

Parenting is one of the most rewarding yet challenging tasks in life. It's filled with beautiful moments of joy and love, but also with uncertainties, pressures, and inevitable chaos. The practice of mindful parenting, empowered by grounding techniques, can help parents navigate this intricate journey with more calmness, clarity, and connection. In this article, we delve into the concept of mindful parenting, the grounding practices that can enhance it, and how these combined approaches can uplift family relationships.

Understanding Mindful Parenting

Mindful parenting involves bringing conscious awareness to the parent-child relationship. It is an ongoing practice that calls for parents to cultivate mindfulness, bringing an open, accepting and non-judgmental presence to interactions with their children. This includes focusing on the present moment, listening with full attention, responding rather than reacting, and recognizing each child's unique individuality. Mindful parenting encourages a warm, understanding, and balanced family environment, which in turn fosters the development of secure, confident, and empathetic children.

Grounding: An Essential Companion to Mindful Parenting

Grounding, also known as earthing, is a practice that aims to reconnect humans with the Earth's natural electric charge. By having direct skin contact with the earth's surface, like walking barefoot in the grass, it's believed that we absorb the Earth's negative electrons, promoting various health benefits such as improved sleep, reduced stress, and increased calmness. Grounding provides an accessible and powerful tool that can be incorporated into a mindful parenting approach.

The Intersection of Grounding and Mindful Parenting

The practices of grounding and mindful parenting are complementary, each enhancing the other's impact on fostering healthy family dynamics. Here's how they intersect.

Promoting Calmness: Parenting can be fraught with high-stress situations. Grounding can help parents manage these stressors, as it has been found to induce physiological changes that promote relaxation. This calm state of mind can then enable a more mindful approach to parenting, allowing parents to respond thoughtfully to their child's needs.

Encouraging Presence: Mindful parenting is rooted in the present moment. Grounding exercises, by nature, bring individuals into the present by focusing their awareness on their connection with the earth. This enhances the ability to be fully present and attentive in interactions with children, a crucial element of mindful parenting.

Modeling Healthy Coping Mechanisms: When parents use grounding techniques to manage their stress and maintain their calm, they inadvertently model healthy coping strategies for their children. This is an essential part of mindful parenting, which encourages the development of emotional regulation skills in children.

Incorporating Grounding into Mindful Parenting

Parents can start incorporating grounding into their parenting routine by spending a few minutes each day connecting with the earth. This could involve walking barefoot in the backyard, gardening, or just sitting outdoors and focusing on the sensations of nature.

These grounding practices can also be shared with children as a family activity, offering an excellent opportunity to teach them about mindfulness and the importance of being present. Children often learn more from what they observe than from what they're told, and seeing their parents routinely practicing grounding can instill in them the value of this practice.

Moreover, parents can apply the calmness and presence they gain from grounding to their everyday interactions with their children. For example, when a child is upset, instead of reacting impulsively, parents can pause, ground themselves, and address the situation with greater calmness and understanding.

Conclusion

Grounding and mindful parenting make a potent combination that can greatly enhance family relationships. Grounding techniques offer an accessible way for parents to cultivate calmness, presence, and patience, key ingredients for mindful parenting. By fostering these qualities, parents can not only enrich their own wellbeing but also create a nurturing, empathetic, and attentive environment that encourages their children's holistic growth. Ultimately, the practice of grounding and mindful parenting reminds us that in the whirlwind of parenting responsibilities, the most profound moments often reside in the here and now, waiting to be cherished.

84. GROUNDING AND THE POWER OF MINDFUL LEADERSHIP

Investigating how Grounding practices can support mindful leadership and enhance workplace culture.

In an era of increasing workplace stress and rapid changes, the need for mindful leadership has never been more critical. Mindful leaders exhibit increased emotional intelligence, self-awareness, and the ability to effectively manage stress and foster resilience within their teams. Grounding techniques can serve as powerful tools in cultivating these qualities and promoting a healthy workplace culture. This article delves into the concepts of mindful leadership and grounding, exploring how these practices intertwine and how they can elevate organizational wellbeing and success.

Understanding Mindful Leadership

Mindful leadership involves the application of mindfulness principles in a leadership context. Mindfulness is the practice of paying attention to the present moment in a non-judgmental manner. Mindful leaders are thus self-aware, conscious of their emotions, and capable of managing them effectively. They can stay focused under pressure, make thoughtful decisions, build strong relationships, and foster a culture of respect, creativity, and resilience.

The Role of Grounding in Mindful Leadership

Grounding, also known as earthing, involves direct physical contact with the Earth's surface (like walking barefoot in the grass or soil) to absorb the Earth's electrons. It's a practice believed to promote various physical and mental health benefits such as stress reduction, improved sleep, and increased calmness. Grounding serves as a practical tool for mindful leaders to nurture their own wellbeing and to enhance their capacity for mindful leadership.

Grounding and Mindful Leadership: A Powerful Synergy

The benefits of grounding practices and mindful leadership can intersect and amplify one another in several ways.

Enhanced Emotional Regulation: Leaders often face high-stress situations that can trigger strong emotional responses. Grounding practices can aid in emotional regulation by inducing relaxation and reducing anxiety. This equips leaders to navigate stressful circumstances with greater calmness and clarity, a key aspect of mindful leadership.

Increased Presence: One of the cornerstones of mindful leadership is the ability to be fully present and attentive. Grounding exercises, by their nature, encourage presence by focusing awareness on one's physical connection with the earth. This can help leaders stay focused, make better decisions, and engage more effectively with their teams.

Improved Stress Management: Stress can impede a leader's cognitive function, decision-making ability, and interpersonal skills. Grounding can counteract these effects by helping to lower stress levels and increase resilience. This supports the mindful leader's capacity to maintain balance and composure in the face of challenges.

Integrating Grounding Practices into Mindful Leadership

Integrating grounding practices into a mindful leadership approach can be a simple process. Leaders could begin their day with a grounding routine, such as walking barefoot outside or doing grounding meditation. These practices could also be used during the workday to manage stress, enhance focus, or restore energy.

In addition, leaders can encourage a grounding mindset within their teams. This might involve integrating brief grounding exercises into meetings, promoting outdoor breaks, or fostering a culture where mindfulness and grounding practices are valued and encouraged.

Impacts on Workplace Culture

The integration of grounding practices into mindful leadership can significantly impact workplace culture. It can foster a more resilient, mindful, and empathetic leadership style, which in turn can influence the overall work environment. When leaders demonstrate calmness, presence, and emotional balance, these qualities can inspire similar behaviors within their teams. This can enhance team cohesion, employee wellbeing, creativity, and productivity.

Conclusion

Grounding practices offer a practical, accessible tool to support mindful leadership. They provide a means to reduce stress, enhance emotional regulation, and cultivate presence, key attributes of successful and respected leaders. By integrating grounding into their leadership approach, leaders can not only enhance their personal wellbeing and effectiveness but also create a more mindful, resilient, and supportive workplace culture. Ultimately, mindful leadership supported by grounding can drive both individual and organizational success, making it a valuable approach for today's dynamic and challenging work environments.

85. GROUNDING AND THE POWER OF MINDFUL TECHNOLOGY USE

Discussing How Grounding Practices Can Support Mindful Technology Use and Promote Digital Well-Being

In our rapidly digitalizing world, technology permeates almost every aspect of our lives. While the benefits of technology are unquestionable, the downsides - such as digital addiction, constant distraction, and mental health issues - are also becoming increasingly apparent. To navigate this digital landscape with balance and well-being, mindful technology use, supported by grounding practices, offers a valuable strategy. This article explores the intersection of grounding practices and mindful technology use, providing insight into how we can enhance our digital well-being.

The Challenges of Digital Overuse

Digital devices and platforms have fundamentally altered how we communicate, work, and entertain ourselves. However, their constant presence has also given rise to new challenges. Many of us grapple with compulsive checking, inability to focus, and anxiety tied to digital consumption. Digital overuse can lead to physical health issues such as poor posture and eye strain, and mental health problems like anxiety, depression, and sleep disorders.

Mindful Technology Use

Mindful technology use is an antidote to these challenges. It involves bringing awareness and intention to our interactions with digital devices and platforms. This may mean limiting time spent on certain applications, taking regular digital detoxes, or simply bringing more presence to our digital interactions. Mindful technology use enables us to leverage technology's benefits without falling prey to its potential harms.

Grounding and Mindful Technology Use

Grounding, also known as earthing, is a therapeutic technique that involves making direct physical contact with the earth to balance the body's electrical energy. It has been associated with a host of health benefits including reduced stress, improved sleep, and increased mental clarity. Grounding practices can play a crucial role in supporting mindful technology use and promoting digital well-being.

Here's how grounding can help us use technology more mindfully.

Promoting Presence: Grounding practices can cultivate a sense of presence, pulling us out of the digital realm and back into the physical world. By fostering a deeper connection with our bodies and the earth, grounding can help us disconnect from our devices and become more present in our daily lives.

Reducing Stress and Anxiety: Grounding has been shown to reduce stress and anxiety, common byproducts of digital overuse. By integrating grounding practices into our routines, we can counterbalance the stress of the digital world and restore a sense of calm and balance.

Enhancing Sleep Quality: Overuse of digital devices, especially before bedtime, can interfere with sleep. Grounding practices can improve sleep quality, counteracting the negative effects of digital consumption on sleep patterns.

Practical Ways to Combine Grounding and Mindful Technology Use

Bringing together grounding and mindful technology use can be achieved through a few practical steps.

Digital Detox Breaks: Regularly disconnect from technology to engage in grounding activities, such as walking barefoot on the grass, meditating outdoors, or gardening.

Mindful Notifications: Use reminders to prompt grounding exercises throughout the day. For example, set a reminder every hour to take a few minutes to practice grounding by focusing on your physical sensations and surroundings.

Tech-Free Zones: Create designated areas in your home where technology is not allowed. Use these spaces for grounding practices, like yoga, meditation, or simply enjoying quiet time.

Conclusion

While technology offers numerous benefits, it also presents challenges that can impact our physical and mental well-being. By combining mindful technology use with grounding practices, we can navigate the digital landscape with more balance, presence, and intention. This fusion of grounding and mindful tech use can serve as a vital tool for maintaining and enhancing our digital well-being in an increasingly tech-dominated world.

HERE IS A LIST OF ILLNESSES THAT GROUNDING MAY POTENTIALLY BE BENEFICIAL

How Grounding Can Help with Mental Health Illnesses

Grounding, or earthing, is the practice of connecting your body to the Earth. This can be done by walking barefoot outside, sitting on the ground, or using a grounding mat or sheet. Grounding has been shown to have a number of health benefits, including:

- Reducing inflammation
- Improving circulation
- Reducing stress
- Balancing hormones
- Boosting the immune system

These benefits can be helpful for a variety of mental health illnesses, including those you listed:

Pain

Aching muscles

Mean: Pain in the muscles that is often dull and aching.

Grounding: Grounding can help to relieve aching muscles by reducing inflammation and oxidative stress. Additionally, grounding can help to improve circulation and reduce muscle tension.

Acute pain

Mean: Short-term pain that is caused by an injury or illness.

Grounding: Grounding can help to reduce acute pain by reducing inflammation and oxidative stress. Additionally, grounding can help to improve circulation and reduce muscle tension.

Arthritis pain

Mean: Pain in the joints that is caused by inflammation.

Grounding: Grounding can help to reduce arthritis pain by reducing inflammation and oxidative stress in the joints. Additionally, grounding can help to improve circulation and reduce joint stiffness.

Back pain

Mean: Pain in the back that can be caused by a variety of factors, such as muscle strain, ligament injury, or disc herniation.

Grounding: Grounding can help to reduce back pain by reducing inflammation and muscle tension in the back. Additionally, grounding can help to improve circulation and reduce muscle spasms.

Burning mouth syndrome

Mean: A condition that causes a burning sensation in the mouth, even when there is no underlying medical condition.

Grounding: Grounding may help to reduce the symptoms of burning mouth syndrome by reducing inflammation and oxidative stress in the mouth. Additionally, grounding may help to improve blood flow to the mouth and reduce nerve sensitivity.

Carpal tunnel syndrome

Mean: A condition that causes numbness, tingling, and weakness in the hand and fingers due to compression of the median nerve.

Grounding: Grounding may help to reduce the symptoms of carpal tunnel syndrome by reducing inflammation and swelling in the wrist. Additionally, grounding may help to improve circulation and nerve function in the hand and fingers.

Chronic pain

Mean: Pain that lasts for more than 12 weeks.

Grounding: Grounding can help to reduce chronic pain by reducing inflammation and oxidative stress in the body. Additionally, grounding can help to improve circulation and reduce muscle tension.

Fibromyalgia pain

Mean: Pain that is widespread throughout the body and is accompanied by other symptoms, such as fatigue, sleep problems, and cognitive impairment.

Grounding: Grounding can help to reduce fibromyalgia pain by reducing inflammation and oxidative stress in the body. Additionally, grounding can help to improve sleep quality and reduce fatigue.

Headaches

Mean: Pain in the head that can be caused by a variety of factors, such as stress, migraines, and tension headaches.

Grounding: Grounding can help to reduce headaches by reducing inflammation and muscle tension in the head and neck. Additionally, grounding may help to improve circulation and reduce stress levels.

Joint pain

Mean: Pain in the joints that can be caused by a variety of factors, such as arthritis, injuries, and infections.

Grounding: Grounding can help to reduce joint pain by reducing inflammation and oxidative stress in the joints. Additionally, grounding can help to improve circulation and reduce joint stiffness.

Menstrual cramps

Mean: Pain in the lower abdomen that occurs during menstruation.

Grounding: Grounding may help to reduce menstrual cramps by reducing inflammation and muscle tension in the abdomen. Additionally, grounding may help to improve circulation and reduce stress levels.

Muscle cramps

Mean: Sudden, involuntary contractions of a muscle.

Grounding: Grounding may help to reduce muscle cramps by improving circulation and reducing muscle tension. Additionally, grounding may help to improve electrolyte balance, which can also help to reduce muscle cramps.

Muscle pain

Mean: Pain in the muscles that can be caused by a variety of factors, such as muscle strain, injury, or overuse.

Grounding: Grounding can help to reduce muscle pain by reducing inflammation and muscle tension. Additionally, grounding can help to improve circulation and reduce muscle spasms.

Muscle soreness

Mean: Pain and discomfort in the muscles that occurs after exercise.

Grounding: Grounding may help to reduce muscle soreness by reducing inflammation and oxidative stress in the muscles. Additionally, grounding may help to improve circulation and reduce muscle tension.

Muscle tension

Mean: Tightness and stiffness in the muscles.

Grounding: Grounding can help to reduce muscle tension by improving circulation and reducing inflammation. Additionally, grounding may help to improve nerve function and relaxation.

Myofascial pain syndrome

Mean: A condition that causes pain, tenderness, and stiffness in the muscles and fascia, which is the connective tissue that surrounds the muscles.

Grounding: Grounding may help to reduce the symptoms of myofascial pain syndrome by reducing inflammation and muscle tension. Additionally, grounding may help to improve circulation and nerve function.

Myositis

Mean: Inflammation of the muscles.

Grounding: Grounding may help to reduce the symptoms of myositis by reducing inflammation and muscle tension. Additionally, grounding may help to improve circulation and nerve function.

Nerve pain

Mean: Pain that is caused by damage or irritation to a nerve.

Grounding: Grounding may help to reduce nerve pain by reducing inflammation and oxidative stress in the nerves. Additionally, grounding may help to improve nerve function and regeneration.

Neuralgia

Mean: Pain that is caused by irritation or damage to a nerve.

Grounding: Grounding may help to reduce neuralgia pain by reducing inflammation and oxidative stress in the nerves. Additionally, grounding may help to improve nerve function and regeneration.

Neuritis

Mean: Inflammation of a nerve.

Grounding: Grounding may help to reduce neuritis pain by reducing inflammation and oxidative stress in the nerves.

Additionally, grounding may help to improve nerve function and regeneration.

Neuropathy

Mean: Damage to the nerves that can cause pain, numbness, and tingling.

Grounding: Grounding may help to reduce neuropathy pain by reducing inflammation and oxidative stress in the nerves. Additionally, grounding may help to improve nerve function and regeneration.

Night terrors

Mean: A sleep disorder that causes children to wake up terrified and screaming.

Grounding: Grounding may help to reduce the frequency and severity of night terrors by reducing stress and anxiety. Additionally, grounding may help to improve sleep quality

Nightmares

Mean: Vivid, disturbing dreams.

Grounding: Grounding may help to reduce the frequency and severity of nightmares by reducing stress and anxiety. Additionally, grounding may help to improve sleep quality.

Pain is associated with autoimmune diseases, such as lupus and rheumatoid arthritis.

Mean: Pain that is caused by inflammation and damage to the tissues and organs in the body.

Grounding: Grounding may help to reduce pain associated with autoimmune diseases by reducing inflammation and oxidative stress. Additionally, grounding may help to improve circulation and nerve function.

Phantom limb pain

Mean: Pain that is felt in a limb that has been amputated.

Grounding: Grounding may help to reduce phantom limb pain by reducing inflammation and oxidative stress in the nervous system. Additionally, grounding may help to improve nerve function and coordination.

Plantar fasciitis

Mean: Inflammation of the plantar fascia, a thick band of tissue that runs along the bottom of the foot.

Grounding: Grounding may help to reduce pain and inflammation in people with plantar fasciitis. This is because grounding can help to improve circulation and reduce inflammation. Additionally, grounding may help to relax the muscles in the feet and calves.

Postherpetic neuralgia

Mean: A type of nerve pain that can occur after an outbreak of shingles.

Grounding: Grounding may help to reduce postherpetic neuralgia pain by reducing inflammation and oxidative stress in the nerves. Additionally, grounding may help to improve nerve function and regeneration.

Post-surgical pain

Mean: Pain that is experienced after surgery.

Grounding: Grounding may help to reduce post-surgical pain by reducing inflammation and oxidative stress. Additionally, grounding may help to improve circulation and reduce muscle spasms.

Raynaud's Syndrome

Mean: A condition that causes the blood vessels in the fingers and toes to narrow in response to cold or stress.

Grounding: Grounding may help to improve circulation in the fingers and toes in people with Raynaud's Syndrome. This is because grounding can help to widen the blood vessels. Additionally, grounding may help to reduce inflammation and oxidative stress, which can also contribute to Raynaud's Syndrome.

Reflex sympathetic dystrophy

Mean: A chronic pain condition that is characterized by pain, burning, and swelling in the extremities.

Grounding: Grounding may help to reduce pain and inflammation in people with reflex sympathetic dystrophy. This is because grounding can help to improve circulation and reduce inflammation. Additionally, grounding may help to relax the muscles and nerves in the extremities.

Restless Legs Syndrome (RLS)

Mean: A neurological disorder that causes an urge to move the legs, especially at night or when sitting for long periods of time.

Grounding: Grounding may help to reduce the symptoms of RLS, such as the urge to move the legs and restlessness. This is because grounding can help to reduce inflammation and oxidative stress in the nervous system. Additionally, grounding may help to improve sleep quality and reduce fatigue.

Sciatica

Mean: Pain that radiates down the leg from the lower back.

Grounding: Grounding may help to reduce sciatica pain by reducing inflammation and muscle tension in the lower back and legs. Additionally, grounding may help to improve circulation and nerve function.

Shin splints

Mean: Pain in the shins that is caused by overuse.

Grounding: Grounding may help to reduce shin splint pain by reducing inflammation and muscle tension in the shins. Additionally, grounding may help to improve circulation and reduce muscle spasms.

Shingles pain

Mean: Pain that is caused by an outbreak of shingles, a viral infection that causes a painful rash on the skin.

Grounding: Grounding may help to reduce shingles pain by reducing inflammation and oxidative stress in the nerves. Additionally, grounding may help to improve nerve function and regeneration.

Sports injuries

Mean: Injuries that are sustained during sports or other physical activities.

Grounding: Grounding may help to reduce pain and inflammation in people with sports injuries. This is because grounding can help to improve circulation and reduce inflammation. Additionally, grounding may help to relax the muscles and nerves in the injured area.

Stress-related health problems, such as high blood pressure and heart disease

Mean: Health problems that are caused by chronic stress.

Grounding: Grounding may help to reduce stress and improve overall health. This is because grounding can help to reduce inflammation and oxidative stress, which are two major factors that contribute to stress-related health problems. Additionally, grounding may help to improve sleep quality and reduce fatigue.

Stroke

Mean: A sudden interruption of blood flow to the brain that causes damage to brain tissue.

Grounding: Grounding may help to improve circulation and nerve function in people who have had a stroke. Additionally, grounding may help to reduce inflammation and oxidative stress in the brain, which Temporomandibular Joint Disorders (TMJ)

Tendinitis

Mean: Inflammation of a tendon, which is a cord of tissue that connects muscle to bone.

Grounding: Grounding may help to reduce pain and inflammation in people with tendinitis. This is because grounding can help to improve circulation and reduce inflammation. Additionally, grounding may help to relax the muscles and tendons.

Tennis elbow

Mean: A condition that causes pain and inflammation in the elbow due to overuse of the tendons in the forearm.

Grounding: Grounding may help to reduce pain and inflammation in people with tennis elbow. This is because grounding can help to improve circulation and reduce inflammation. Additionally, grounding may help to relax the muscles and tendons in the forearm.

Tonsillitis

Mean: Inflammation of the tonsils, which are two small masses of tissue at the back of the throat.

Grounding: Grounding may help to reduce pain and inflammation in people with tonsillitis. This is because grounding can help to improve circulation and reduce inflammation. Additionally, grounding may help to boost the immune system and fight infection.

Toxic Shock Syndrome

Mean: A rare but serious infection that can be caused by bacteria.

Grounding: Grounding may help to improve circulation and reduce inflammation in people with toxic shock syndrome.

Additionally, grounding may help to boost the immune system and fight infection.

Traumatic Brain Injury

Mean: An injury to the brain that is caused by a sudden impact or jolt.

Grounding: Grounding may help to improve circulation and nerve function in people who have had a traumatic brain injury. Additionally, grounding may help to reduce inflammation and oxidative stress in the brain, which can help to protect the brain from further damage.

Trigeminal neuralgia

Mean: A chronic pain condition that affects the trigeminal nerve, which is a nerve that provides sensation to the face and head.

Grounding: Grounding may help to reduce pain and inflammation in people with trigeminal neuralgia. This is because grounding can help to improve circulation and reduce inflammation. Additionally, grounding may help to relax the muscles and nerves in the face and head.

Ulcerative colitis

Mean: An inflammatory bowel disease that causes inflammation and ulcers in the colon.

Grounding: Grounding may help to reduce inflammation and oxidative stress in the colon, which are two major factors that contribute to ulcerative colitis. Additionally, grounding may help to improve gut health and digestion.

Ulcers

Mean: Sores that can form on the lining of the stomach or intestines.

Grounding: Grounding may help to reduce inflammation and oxidative stress in the stomach and intestines, which are two major factors that contribute to ulcers. Additionally, grounding may help to improve circulation and promote healing.

Urinary Tract Infections (UTIs)

Mean: Infections in any part of the urinary system, including the kidneys, bladder, or urethra.

Grounding: Grounding may help to reduce inflammation and oxidative stress in the urinary system, which can help to prevent and treat UTIs. Additionally, grounding may help to improve circulation and boost the immune system.

Varicose Veins

Mean: Swollen veins that bulge just below the skin.

Grounding: Grounding may help to improve circulation in the legs and reduce the severity of varicose veins. This is because grounding can help to widen the blood vessels and improve valve function. Additionally, grounding may help to reduce inflammation and oxidative stress, which can also contribute to varicose veins.

Vertigo

Mean: A feeling of dizziness or spinning.

Grounding: Grounding may help to reduce vertigo by improving circulation and balance. Additionally, grounding may help to reduce stress and anxiety, which can also contribute to vertigo.

Wound healing

Mean: The process of repairing damaged tissue.

Grounding: Grounding may help to improve wound healing by increasing blood flow to the injured area and reducing inflammation. Additionally, grounding may help to promote the growth of new tissue.

Inflammation

Acne

Mean: A skin condition that causes pimples, blackheads, and whiteheads.

Grounding: Grounding may help to reduce acne by reducing inflammation and oxidative stress in the skin. Additionally, grounding may help to improve circulation and boost the immune system.

Allergies

Mean: An overreaction of the immune system to a harmless substance, such as pollen, dust mites, or pet dander.

Grounding: Grounding may help to reduce allergies by reducing inflammation and oxidative stress in the body. Additionally, grounding may help to improve circulation and boost the immune system.

Arthritis

Mean: A condition that causes pain, inflammation, and stiffness in the joints.

Grounding: Grounding may help to reduce arthritis pain and inflammation by reducing inflammation and oxidative stress in the joints. Additionally, grounding may help to improve circulation and reduce muscle tension.

Asthma

Mean: A chronic lung disease that causes inflammation and narrowing of the airways.

Grounding: Grounding may help to improve asthma symptoms by reducing inflammation and oxidative stress in the airways. Additionally, grounding may help to relax the muscles in the airways and improve breathing.

Atherosclerosis

Mean: A condition in which plaque builds up on the walls of the arteries, narrowing them and restricting blood flow.

Grounding: Grounding may help to reduce the risk of atherosclerosis by reducing inflammation and oxidative stress in the arteries. Additionally, grounding may help to improve circulation and widen the blood vessels.

Autoimmune diseases, such as lupus and rheumatoid arthritis

Mean: Diseases in which the body's immune system attacks its own tissues.

Grounding: Grounding may help to reduce the symptoms of autoimmune diseases by reducing inflammation and oxidative stress in the body. Additionally, grounding may help to improve circulation and boost the immune system.

Chronic Inflammatory Conditions

Mean: Conditions that are characterized by inflammation, such as inflammatory bowel disease, psoriasis, and multiple sclerosis.

Grounding: Grounding may help to reduce the symptoms of chronic inflammatory conditions by reducing inflammation and oxidative stress in the body. Additionally, grounding may help to improve circulation and boost the immune system.

Colon Polyps

Mean: Growths on the lining of the colon that can turn into cancer if not removed.

Grounding: Grounding may help to reduce the risk of colon polyps by reducing inflammation and oxidative stress in the colon. Additionally, grounding may help to improve digestion and promote gut health.

Common cold

Mean: A viral infection of the upper respiratory tract that causes symptoms such as sneezing, runny nose, and sore throat.

Grounding: Grounding may help to reduce the symptoms of the common cold by reducing inflammation and oxidative stress in the body. Additionally, grounding may help to boost the immune system and fight infection.

Crohn's disease

Mean: An inflammatory bowel disease that causes inflammation and ulcers in the digestive tract.

Grounding: Grounding may help to reduce inflammation and oxidative stress in the digestive tract, which are two major factors that contribute to Crohn's disease. Additionally, grounding may help to improve gut health and digestion.

Cystitis

Mean: Inflammation of the bladder.

Grounding: Grounding may help to reduce inflammation and oxidative stress in the bladder. Additionally, grounding may help to boost the immune system and fight infection.

Decompression Sickness

Mean: A condition caused by rapid changes in pressure, such as when diving or flying.

Grounding: Grounding may help to reduce the symptoms of decompression sickness by improving circulation and reducing inflammation.

Dermatitis

Mean: Inflammation of the skin.

Grounding: Grounding may help to reduce inflammation and oxidative stress in the skin. Additionally, grounding may help to improve circulation and boost the immune system.

Eczema

Mean: A chronic skin condition that causes dry, itchy skin.

Grounding: Grounding may help to reduce the symptoms of eczema by reducing inflammation and oxidative stress in the skin. Additionally, grounding may help to improve circulation and boost the immune system.

Endometriosis

Mean: A condition in which the tissue that lines the uterus grows outside of the uterus.

Grounding: Grounding may help to reduce the symptoms of endometriosis by reducing inflammation and oxidative stress. Additionally, grounding may help to improve circulation and reduce muscle tension.

Food Allergies

Mean: An overreaction of the immune system to a food protein.

Grounding: Grounding may help to reduce the symptoms of food allergies by reducing inflammation and oxidative stress in the body. Additionally, grounding may help to improve circulation and boost the immune system.

Food Sensitivities

Mean: A negative reaction to a food that does not involve the immune system.

Grounding: Grounding may help to reduce the symptoms of food sensitivities by reducing inflammation and oxidative stress in the body. Additionally, grounding may help to improve circulation and boost the immune system.

Gallstones

Mean: Solid stones that form in the gallbladder.

Grounding: Grounding may help to reduce the risk of gallstones by improving digestion and gallbladder function. Additionally, grounding may help to reduce inflammation and oxidative stress in the gallbladder.

Gastritis

Mean: Inflammation of the lining of the stomach.

Grounding: Grounding may help to reduce inflammation and oxidative stress in the stomach. Additionally, grounding may help to improve circulation and digestion.

Gastroesophageal Reflux Disease (GERD)

Mean: A condition in which stomach acid backs up into the esophagus.

Grounding: Grounding may help to reduce the symptoms of GERD by reducing inflammation and oxidative stress in the esophagus. Additionally, grounding may help to improve digestion and reduce muscle tension in the lower esophageal sphincter.

Gout

Mean: A type of arthritis that causes inflammation and pain in the joints, especially the big toe.

Grounding: Grounding may help to reduce gout pain and inflammation by reducing inflammation and oxidative stress in the joints. Additionally, grounding may help to improve circulation and reduce muscle tension.

Grave's disease

Mean: An autoimmune disease that causes the thyroid gland to produce too much thyroid hormone.

Grounding: Grounding may help to reduce the symptoms of Grave's disease by reducing inflammation and oxidative stress in the body. Additionally, grounding may help to improve circulation and boost the immune system.

Gum Diseases

Mean: Infections and inflammation of the gums and supporting tissues.

Grounding: Grounding may help to reduce inflammation and oxidative stress in the gums. Additionally, grounding may help to improve circulation and boost the immune system.

Hashimoto's Thyroiditis

Mean: An autoimmune disease that causes the thyroid gland to be underactive.

Grounding: Grounding may help to improve the symptoms of Hashimoto's thyroiditis by reducing inflammation and oxidative stress in the body. Additionally, grounding may help to improve circulation and boost the immune system.

Hay Fever

Mean: An allergic reaction to pollen.

Grounding: Grounding may help to reduce the symptoms of hay fever by reducing inflammation and oxidative stress in the body. Additionally, grounding may help to improve circulation and boost the immune system.

Inflammation

Mean: A biological response to injury or infection that is characterized by pain, swelling, heat, and redness.

Grounding: Grounding may help to reduce inflammation by reducing inflammation and oxidative stress in the body. Additionally, grounding may help to improve circulation and reduce muscle tension.

Influenza

Mean: A viral infection of the respiratory system that causes fever, cough, sore throat, and muscle aches.

Grounding: Grounding may help to reduce the symptoms of influenza by reducing inflammation and oxidative stress in the body. Additionally, grounding may help to boost the immune system and fight infection.

Grounding: Grounding may help to reduce the symptoms of interstitial cystitis by reducing inflammation and oxidative stress in the bladder. Additionally, grounding may help to improve circulation and reduce muscle tension in the bladder.

Irritable bowel syndrome (IBS)

Mean: A chronic disorder that affects the colon and causes symptoms such as abdominal pain, cramping, bloating, and diarrhea.

Grounding: Grounding may help to reduce the symptoms of IBS by reducing inflammation and oxidative stress in the colon. Additionally, grounding may help to improve digestion and reduce muscle tension in the colon.

Laryngitis

Mean: Inflammation of the larynx, or voice box.

Grounding: Grounding may help to reduce inflammation and oxidative stress in the larynx. Additionally, grounding may help to improve circulation and reduce muscle tension in the larynx.

Lupus (SLE)

Mean: An autoimmune disease that can cause inflammation and damage to any part of the body.

Grounding: Grounding may help to reduce the symptoms of lupus by reducing inflammation and oxidative stress in the body. Additionally, grounding may help to improve circulation and boost the immune system.

Lyme disease

Mean: A bacterial infection transmitted by ticks that can cause a variety of symptoms, including fever, headache, rash, and joint pain.

Grounding: Grounding may help to reduce the symptoms of Lyme disease by reducing inflammation and oxidative stress in the body. Additionally, grounding may help to improve circulation and boost the immune system.

Menstrual cramps

Mean: Pain in the lower abdomen that occurs during menstruation.

Grounding: Grounding may help to reduce menstrual cramps by reducing inflammation and muscle tension in the abdomen. Additionally, grounding may help to improve circulation and reduce stress levels.

Multiple sclerosis

Mean: An autoimmune disease that affects the central nervous system.

Grounding: Grounding may help to improve the symptoms of multiple sclerosis by reducing inflammation and oxidative stress in the central nervous system. Additionally, grounding may help to improve circulation and nerve function.

Myositis

Mean: Inflammation of the muscles.

Grounding: Grounding may help to reduce myositis pain and inflammation by reducing inflammation and oxidative stress in the muscles. Additionally, grounding may help to improve circulation and reduce muscle tension.

Osteoarthritis

Mean: A type of arthritis that causes the cartilage in the joints to break down.

Grounding: Grounding may help to reduce osteoarthritis pain and inflammation by reducing inflammation and oxidative stress in the joints. Additionally, grounding may help to improve circulation and reduce muscle tension.

Peptic Ulcer Disease

Mean: Sores that develop on the lining of the stomach or duodenum.

Grounding: Grounding may help to reduce the symptoms of peptic ulcer disease by reducing inflammation and oxidative stress in the stomach and duodenum. Additionally, grounding may help to improve circulation and promote healing.

PMDD (Premenstrual Dysphoric Disorder)

Mean: A mood disorder that occurs in the week or two before menstruation.

Grounding: Grounding may help to improve the symptoms of PMDD by reducing inflammation and oxidative stress in the body. Additionally, grounding may help to improve.

PMS (Premenstrual Syndrome)

Mean: A group of symptoms that occur in the week or two before menstruation.

Grounding: Grounding may help to improve the symptoms of PMS by reducing inflammation and oxidative stress in the body.

Additionally, grounding may help to improve circulation and reduce stress levels.

Pneumonia

Mean: An infection of the lungs that causes inflammation and difficulty breathing.

Grounding: Grounding may help to improve the symptoms of pneumonia by reducing inflammation and oxidative stress in the lungs. Additionally, grounding may help to improve circulation and boost the immune system.

Polycystic Ovary Syndrome (PCOS)

Mean: A hormonal disorder that can cause infertility, acne, and excessive hair growth.

Grounding: Grounding may help to improve the symptoms of PCOS by reducing inflammation and oxidative stress in the body. Additionally, grounding may help to improve circulation and boost the immune system.

Psoriasis

Mean: A chronic skin condition that causes red, itchy patches of skin covered with silvery scales.

Grounding: Grounding may help to reduce the symptoms of psoriasis by reducing inflammation and oxidative stress in the skin. Additionally, grounding may help to improve circulation and boost the immune system.

Psoriatic arthritis

Mean: A type of arthritis that affects people with psoriasis.

Grounding: Grounding may help to reduce the symptoms of psoriatic arthritis by reducing inflammation and oxidative stress in the joints. Additionally, grounding may help to improve circulation and reduce muscle tension.

Rheumatoid arthritis

Mean: An autoimmune disease that causes inflammation and damage to the joints.

Grounding: Grounding may help to reduce rheumatoid arthritis pain and inflammation by reducing inflammation and oxidative stress in the joints. Additionally, grounding may help to improve circulation and reduce muscle tension.

Scleroderma

Mean: A chronic autoimmune disease that causes hardening and thickening of the skin and connective tissues.

Grounding: Grounding may help to improve the symptoms of scleroderma by reducing inflammation and oxidative stress in the body. Additionally, grounding may help to improve circulation and reduce muscle tension.

Shingles

Mean: A viral infection that causes a painful rash on the skin.

Grounding: Grounding may help to reduce the symptoms of shingles by reducing inflammation and oxidative stress in the skin. Additionally, grounding may help to improve circulation and boost the immune system.

Skin conditions, such as eczema and psoriasis

Mean: Conditions that cause inflammation and irritation of the skin.

Grounding: Grounding may help to reduce the symptoms of skin conditions such as eczema and psoriasis by reducing inflammation and oxidative stress in the skin. Additionally, grounding may help to improve circulation and boost the immune system.

Tendinitis

Mean: Inflammation of a tendon, which is a cord of tissue that connects muscle to bone.

Grounding: Grounding may help to reduce tendinitis pain and inflammation by reducing inflammation and oxidative stress in the tendons. Additionally, grounding may help to improve circulation and reduce muscle tension.

Ulcerative colitis

Mean: An inflammatory bowel disease that causes inflammation and ulcers in the colon.

Grounding: Grounding may help to reduce the symptoms of ulcerative colitis by reducing inflammation and oxidative stress in the colon. Additionally, grounding may help to improve digestion and reduce muscle tension in the colon.

Stress and Anxiety

Anxiety disorders

Mean: A group of mental health disorders that cause excessive nervousness, fear, anxiety, and worry.

Grounding: Grounding can help to reduce anxiety symptoms by calming the nervous system and promoting relaxation. Additionally, grounding can help to focus the mind on the present moment and reduce rumination and negative thoughts.

Depression

Mean: A mood disorder that causes persistent feelings of sadness and loss of interest.

Grounding: Grounding can help to improve mood and reduce depressive symptoms by promoting relaxation, increasing self-awareness, and reducing negative thoughts. Additionally, grounding can help to improve sleep quality and increase energy levels.

Erectile Dysfunction

Mean: A sexual dysfunction that causes difficulty getting or maintaining an erection.

Grounding: Grounding can help to improve erectile dysfunction by reducing stress and anxiety, which are two common causes of the condition. Additionally, grounding can help to improve circulation and increase blood flow to the penis.

Generalized anxiety disorder (GAD)

Mean: A type of anxiety disorder that causes excessive worry about a variety of events or activities.

Grounding: Grounding can be an effective way to reduce anxiety symptoms in people with GAD. Grounding can help to calm the nervous system, focus the mind on the present moment, and reduce rumination and negative thoughts.

Obsessive-compulsive disorder (OCD)

Mean: A mental health disorder that causes unwanted and intrusive thoughts (obsessions) and repetitive behaviors or rituals (compulsions).

Grounding: Grounding can be an effective way to manage OCD symptoms. Grounding can help to reduce anxiety, focus the mind on the present moment, and reduce rumination and negative thoughts. Additionally, grounding can help to break the cycle of obsessions and compulsions.

Panic disorder

Mean: A type of anxiety disorder that causes sudden and unexpected panic attacks.

Grounding: Grounding can be an effective way to reduce the frequency and severity of panic attacks. Grounding can help to calm the nervous system, focus the mind on the present moment, and reduce rumination and negative thoughts. Additionally, grounding can help to develop coping skills for managing panic attacks.

Postpartum depression

Mean: A type of depression that can occur after childbirth.

Grounding: Grounding can be an effective way to reduce the symptoms of postpartum depression. Grounding can help to promote relaxation, reduce stress and anxiety, and improve mood. Additionally, grounding can help to connect mothers with their babies and improve the mother-infant bond.

Post-traumatic stress disorder (PTSD)

Mean: A mental health disorder that can develop after exposure to a traumatic event.

Grounding: Grounding can be an effective way to manage PTSD symptoms. Grounding can help to reduce anxiety and flashbacks, and focus the mind on the present moment. Additionally, grounding can help to develop coping skills for managing PTSD symptoms.

Seasonal affective disorder (SAD)

Mean: A type of depression that occurs during the winter months.

Grounding: Grounding can be an effective way to improve mood and reduce depressive symptoms in people with SAD. Grounding can help to promote relaxation, reduce stress and anxiety, and increase energy levels. Additionally, grounding can help to improve sleep quality.

Social anxiety disorder

Mean: A type of anxiety disorder that causes excessive fear or anxiety in social situations.

Grounding: Grounding can be an effective way to reduce anxiety symptoms in people with social anxiety disorder. Grounding can help to calm the nervous system, focus the mind on the present moment, and reduce rumination and negative thoughts. Additionally, grounding can help to develop coping skills for managing social anxiety.

Stress

Mean: A state of mental or emotional strain or tension resulting from adverse or demanding circumstances.

Grounding: Grounding can be an effective way to reduce stress and promote relaxation. Grounding can help to calm the nervous system, focus the mind on the present moment, and reduce negative thoughts. Additionally, grounding can help to improve sleep quality and increase energy levels.

Immune Function

Allergies

Mean: An overreaction of the immune system to a harmless substance, such as pollen, dust mites, or pet dander.

Grounding: Grounding may help to reduce allergies by reducing inflammation and oxidative stress in the body. Additionally, grounding may help to improve circulation and boost the immune system.

Autoimmune diseases

Mean: Diseases in which the body's immune system attacks its own tissues.

Grounding: Grounding may help to reduce the symptoms of autoimmune diseases by reducing inflammation and oxidative stress in the body. Additionally, grounding may help to improve circulation and boost the immune system.

Chronic infections

Mean: Infections that last for more than three months.

Grounding: Grounding may help to reduce the symptoms of chronic infections by boosting the immune system and reducing inflammation. Additionally, grounding may help to improve circulation and promote healing.

Common cold

Mean: A viral infection of the upper respiratory tract that causes symptoms such as sneezing, runny nose, and sore throat.

Grounding: Grounding may help to reduce the symptoms of the common cold by boosting the immune system and reducing inflammation. Additionally, grounding may help to improve circulation and promote healing.

Epstein-Barr virus

Mean: A virus that causes mononucleosis, a condition characterized by fever, sore throat, and swollen lymph glands.

Grounding: Grounding may help to reduce the symptoms of Epstein-Barr virus infection by boosting the immune system and reducing inflammation. Additionally, grounding may help to improve circulation and promote healing.

HIV/AIDS

Mean: A viral infection that attacks the immune system and can lead to AIDS.

Grounding: Grounding may help to improve the immune system and reduce inflammation in people with HIV/AIDS. Additionally, grounding may help to reduce stress and improve sleep quality.

Immune System Disorders

Mean: Conditions that affect the immune system, making it difficult for the body to fight off infection.

Grounding: Grounding may help to improve the immune system and reduce inflammation in people with immune system disorders. Additionally, grounding may help to reduce stress and improve sleep quality.

Lupus

Mean: An autoimmune disease that can cause inflammation and damage to any part of the body.

Grounding: Grounding may help to reduce the symptoms of lupus by reducing inflammation and oxidative stress in the body. Additionally, grounding may help to improve circulation and boost the immune system.

Lyme disease

Mean: A bacterial infection transmitted by ticks that can cause a variety of symptoms, including fever, headache, rash, and joint pain.

Grounding: Grounding may help to reduce the symptoms of Lyme disease by boosting the immune system and reducing inflammation. Additionally, grounding may help to improve circulation and promote healing.

Multiple sclerosis

Mean: An autoimmune disease that affects the central nervous system.

Grounding: Grounding may help to improve the symptoms of multiple sclerosis by reducing inflammation and oxidative stress in the central nervous system. Additionally, grounding may help to improve circulation and nerve function.

Pneumonia

Mean: An infection of the lungs that causes inflammation and difficulty breathing.

Grounding: Grounding may help to reduce the symptoms of pneumonia by boosting the immune system and reducing inflammation in the lungs. Additionally, grounding may help to improve circulation and promote healing.

Polycystic Ovary Syndrome (PCOS)

Mean: A hormonal disorder that can cause infertility, acne, and excessive hair growth.

Grounding: Grounding may help to improve the symptoms of PCOS by reducing inflammation and oxidative stress in the body. Additionally, grounding may help to improve circulation and boost the immune system.

Rheumatoid arthritis

Mean: An autoimmune disease that causes inflammation and damage to the joints.

Grounding: Grounding may help to reduce the symptoms of rheumatoid arthritis by reducing inflammation and oxidative stress in the joints. Additionally, grounding may help to improve circulation and reduce muscle tension.

Sickle cell disease

Mean: A blood disorder that causes the red blood cells to become sickle-shaped, which can block blood vessels and cause pain and other complications.

Grounding: Grounding may help to reduce the symptoms of sickle cell disease by improving circulation and reducing inflammation. Additionally, grounding may help to reduce pain and improve sleep quality.

Sjögren's syndrome

Mean: An autoimmune disease that causes dryness of the mouth and eyes.

Grounding: Grounding may help to improve the symptoms of Sjögren's syndrome by reducing inflammation and oxidative stress in the body. Additionally, grounding may help to improve circulation and boost the immune system.

Sleep

Bruxism

Mean: Grinding or clenching of the teeth.

Grounding: Grounding may help to reduce bruxism by reducing stress and anxiety, which are two common triggers of the condition. Additionally, grounding may help to improve relaxation and sleep quality.

Chronic Insomnia

Mean: Difficulty falling asleep and/or staying asleep for more than three months.

Grounding: Grounding may help to improve chronic insomnia by promoting relaxation, reducing stress and anxiety, and regulating the circadian rhythm. Additionally, grounding may help to improve sleep quality.

Circadian rhythm sleep disorder

Mean: A sleep disorder that occurs when the body's internal sleep-wake cycle is disrupted.

Grounding: Grounding may help to improve circadian rhythm sleep disorders by regulating the circadian rhythm and promoting relaxation. Additionally, grounding may help to reduce stress and anxiety, which can interfere with sleep.

Hypersomnia

Mean: Excessive daytime sleepiness.

Grounding: Grounding may help to improve hypersomnia by increasing energy levels and reducing fatigue. Additionally, grounding may help to improve sleep quality at night.

Insomnia

Mean: Difficulty falling asleep and/or staying asleep.

Grounding: Grounding may help to improve insomnia by promoting relaxation, reducing stress and anxiety, and regulating the circadian rhythm. Additionally, grounding may help to improve sleep quality.

Narcolepsy

Mean: A chronic sleep disorder that causes excessive daytime sleepiness, sudden attacks of sleep, and cataplexy (a sudden loss of muscle control triggered by strong emotions).

Grounding: Grounding may help to improve narcolepsy by increasing energy levels and reducing fatigue. Additionally, grounding may help to improve sleep quality at night.

Night Terrors

Mean: Sudden and intense episodes of fear that occur during sleep.

Grounding: Grounding may help to reduce night terrors by promoting relaxation and reducing stress and anxiety. Additionally, grounding may help to improve sleep quality.

Nightmares

Mean: Vivid and disturbing dreams that occur during sleep.

Grounding: Grounding may help to reduce nightmares by promoting relaxation and reducing stress and anxiety. Additionally, grounding may help to improve sleep quality.

Obstructive sleep apnea

Mean: A sleep disorder in which breathing is repeatedly interrupted during sleep.

Grounding: Grounding may help to improve obstructive sleep apnea by reducing inflammation and improving circulation in the airways. Additionally, grounding may help to reduce stress and anxiety, which can worsen the condition.

Sleep apnea

Mean: A sleep disorder in which breathing is repeatedly interrupted during sleep.

Grounding: Grounding may help to improve sleep apnea by reducing inflammation and improving circulation in the airways. Additionally, grounding may help to reduce stress and anxiety, which can worsen the condition.

Sleep Disorders

Mean: A group of conditions that affect sleep.

Grounding: Grounding may help to improve a variety of sleep disorders by promoting relaxation, reducing stress and anxiety, regulating the circadian rhythm, and improving sleep quality.

Sleep-Related Eating Disorders

Mean: Disorders that involve eating or drinking during sleep.

Grounding: Grounding may help to improve sleep-related eating disorders by promoting relaxation, reducing stress and anxiety, and improving sleep quality. Additionally, grounding may help to increase awareness of sleep and reduce sleepwalking.

Sleepwalking

Mean: A sleep disorder in which people walk or perform other complex behaviors while asleep.

Grounding: Grounding may help to improve sleepwalking by increasing awareness of sleep and reducing the frequency of sleepwalking episodes. Additionally, grounding may help to improve sleep quality.

Snoring

Mean: A noisy breathing sound that occurs during sleep.

Grounding: Grounding may help to reduce snoring by reducing inflammation in the airways. Additionally, grounding may help to promote relaxation and improve sleep quality.

Other Conditions

Addison's Disease

Mean: A chronic autoimmune disease that causes the adrenal glands to not produce enough of the hormones cortisol and aldosterone.

Grounding: Grounding may help to improve the symptoms of Addison's disease by reducing inflammation and oxidative stress in the body. Additionally, grounding may help to improve circulation and boost the immune system.

Adenoiditis

Mean: Inflammation of the adenoids, which are two small pads of tissue located at the back of the throat.

Grounding: Grounding may help to reduce the symptoms of adenoiditis by reducing inflammation and oxidative stress in the body. Additionally, grounding may help to improve circulation and boost the immune system.

Adrenal Fatigue

Mean: A condition in which the adrenal glands are unable to produce enough of the hormones cortisol and aldosterone.

Grounding: Grounding may help to improve the symptoms of adrenal fatigue by reducing inflammation and oxidative stress in the body. Additionally, grounding may help to improve circulation and boost the immune system.

Adrenal Insufficiency

Mean: A condition in which the adrenal glands do not produce enough hormones, such as cortisol and aldosterone.

Grounding: Grounding may help to improve the symptoms of adrenal insufficiency by reducing inflammation and oxidative stress in the body. Additionally, grounding may help to improve circulation and boost the immune system.

AIDS/HIV

Mean: A chronic viral infection that attacks the immune system and can lead to AIDS.

Grounding: Grounding may help to improve the immune system and reduce inflammation in people with HIV/AIDS. Additionally, grounding may help to reduce stress and improve sleep quality.

Alcoholism

Mean: A chronic disease characterized by excessive alcohol consumption.

Grounding: Grounding may help to reduce cravings for alcohol and improve mood in people with alcoholism. Additionally, grounding may help to promote relaxation and reduce stress.

Alopecia (Hair Loss)

Mean: A condition characterized by excessive hair loss.

Grounding: Grounding may help to improve hair growth by reducing inflammation and oxidative stress in the scalp. Additionally, grounding may help to improve circulation and boost the immune system.

Altitude Sickness

Mean: A condition caused by exposure to high altitudes.

Grounding: Grounding may help to reduce the symptoms of altitude sickness by improving circulation and oxygen levels in the blood. Additionally, grounding may help to reduce inflammation and oxidative stress in the body.

Alzheimer's Disease

Mean: A chronic neurodegenerative disease that causes progressive memory loss and cognitive decline.

Grounding: Grounding may help to improve cognitive function and reduce the symptoms of Alzheimer's disease by reducing inflammation and oxidative stress in the brain. Additionally, grounding may help to improve circulation and boost the immune system.

Amyotrophic Lateral Sclerosis (ALS)

Mean: A chronic neurodegenerative disease that affects the nerve cells in the brain and spinal cord.

Grounding: Grounding may help to improve muscle function and reduce the symptoms of ALS by reducing inflammation and oxidative stress in the nerves. Additionally, grounding may help to improve circulation and boost the immune system.

Anoxia

Mean: A condition in which the body's tissues do not receive enough oxygen.

Grounding: Grounding may help to improve oxygen levels in the blood and reduce the symptoms of anoxia by improving circulation. Additionally, grounding may help to reduce inflammation and oxidative stress in the body.

Arrhythmias

Mean: Abnormal heart rhythms.

Grounding: Grounding may help to improve heart rate and rhythm by reducing inflammation and oxidative stress in the heart. Additionally, grounding may help to promote relaxation and reduce stress.

Attention deficit hyperactivity disorder (ADHD)

Mean: A neurodevelopmental disorder characterized by inattention, hyperactivity, and impulsivity.

Grounding: Grounding may help to improve attention and focus in people with ADHD by reducing stress and anxiety. Additionally, grounding may help to promote relaxation and improve sleep quality.

Autism Spectrum Disorders

Mean: A group of neurodevelopmental disorders characterized by social communication and interaction challenges, and restricted interests and repetitive behaviors.

Grounding: Grounding may help to improve social communication and interaction skills in people with autism spectrum disorders by reducing stress and anxiety. Additionally, grounding may help to promote relaxation and improve sleep quality.

Bell's Palsy

Mean: A sudden weakness or paralysis on one side of the face.

Grounding: Grounding may help to improve facial muscle function in people with Bell's palsy by reducing inflammation and oxidative stress in the nerves. Additionally, grounding may help to promote relaxation and reduce stress.

Bipolar disorder

Mean: A mental health condition that causes extreme mood swings that include emotional highs (mania or hypomania) and lows (depression).

Grounding: Grounding may help to improve mood stability and reduce the symptoms of bipolar disorder by reducing inflammation and oxidative stress in the brain. Additionally, grounding may help to promote relaxation and reduce stress.

Bone Fractures

Mean: A break in a bone.

Grounding: Grounding may help to promote bone healing and reduce pain in people with bone fractures by improving circulation and reducing inflammation. Additionally, grounding may help to reduce stress and promote relaxation.

Bronchitis

Mean: Inflammation of the bronchi, which are the tubes that carry air to and from the lungs.

Grounding: Grounding may help to reduce the symptoms of bronchitis by reducing inflammation and oxidative stress in the lungs. Additionally, grounding may help to improve circulation and boost the immune system.

Bruxism (Teeth Grinding)

Mean: The grinding or clenching of teeth.

Grounding: Grounding may help to reduce bruxism by reducing stress and anxiety, which are two common triggers of the condition. Additionally, grounding may help to improve relaxation and sleep quality.

Burning mouth syndrome

Mean: A condition characterized by a burning sensation in the mouth without an obvious cause.

Grounding: Grounding may help to reduce the symptoms of burning mouth syndrome by reducing inflammation and oxidative stress in the mouth. Additionally, grounding may help to promote relaxation and reduce stress.

Bursitis

Mean: Inflammation of a bursa, which is a small fluid-filled sac that cushions bones, tendons, and muscles.

Grounding: Grounding may help to reduce inflammation and pain in people with bursitis by reducing inflammation and oxidative stress. Additionally, grounding may help to improve circulation and promote healing.

Cancer

Mean: A disease in which abnormal cells divide uncontrollably and destroy healthy tissue.

Grounding: Grounding may help to improve the quality of life and reduce the side effects of cancer and cancer treatment by reducing inflammation and oxidative stress in the body. Additionally, grounding may help to promote relaxation and reduce stress.

Cardiovascular disease

Mean: A group of diseases that affect the heart and blood vessels.

Grounding: Grounding may help to improve cardiovascular health and reduce the risk of cardiovascular disease by reducing inflammation and oxidative stress in the heart and blood vessels. Additionally, grounding may help to promote relaxation and reduce stress.

Cataracts

Mean: A clouding of the lens of the eye, which can cause blurred vision, difficulty seeing at night, and sensitivity to light.

Grounding: Grounding may help to improve vision and reduce the symptoms of cataracts by reducing inflammation and oxidative stress in the eyes. Additionally, grounding may help to improve circulation and boost the immune system.

Celiac disease

Mean: An autoimmune disease that damages the small intestine when gluten is eaten.

Grounding: Grounding may help to reduce inflammation and oxidative stress in the digestive tract in people with celiac disease. Additionally, grounding may help to improve circulation and boost the immune system.

Cerebral Palsy

Mean: A group of disorders that affect movement and coordination.

Grounding: Grounding may help to improve muscle function and coordination in people with cerebral palsy by reducing inflammation and oxidative stress in the nerves and muscles. Additionally, grounding may help to promote relaxation and reduce stress.

Chronic Edema

Mean: Buildup of fluid in the tissues.

Grounding: Grounding may help to reduce edema by improving circulation and reducing inflammation. Additionally, grounding may help to promote relaxation and reduce stress.

Chronic fatigue syndrome

Mean: A condition characterized by extreme fatigue that cannot be explained by an underlying medical condition.

Grounding: Grounding may help to improve energy levels and reduce fatigue in people with chronic fatigue syndrome by reducing inflammation and oxidative stress in the body. Additionally, grounding may help to promote relaxation and improve sleep quality.

Chronic Hepatitis

Mean: Long-term inflammation of the liver.

Grounding: Grounding may help to reduce inflammation and oxidative stress in the liver in people with chronic hepatitis. Additionally, grounding may help to improve circulation and boost the immune system.

Circulation Problems

Mean: Conditions that affect blood flow throughout the body.

Grounding: Grounding may help to improve circulation by reducing inflammation and oxidative stress in the blood vessels. Additionally, grounding may help to promote relaxation and reduce stress.

Cirrhosis

Mean: A chronic liver disease that causes scarring and damage to the liver.

Grounding: Grounding may help to reduce inflammation and oxidative stress in the liver in people with cirrhosis. Additionally, grounding may help to improve circulation and boost the immune system.

Constipation

Mean: Difficulty passing stool.

Grounding: Grounding may help to improve digestion and reduce constipation by reducing inflammation and oxidative stress in the digestive tract. Additionally, grounding may help to promote relaxation and reduce stress.

COPD (Chronic Obstructive Pulmonary Disease)

Mean: A group of lung diseases that block airflow and make it difficult to breathe.

Grounding: Grounding may help to improve breathing and reduce the symptoms of COPD by reducing inflammation and oxidative stress in the lungs. Additionally, grounding may help to improve circulation and boost the immune system.

Dementia

Mean: A group of conditions that cause progressive memory loss and cognitive decline.

Grounding: Grounding may help to improve cognitive function and reduce the symptoms of dementia by reducing inflammation and oxidative stress in the brain. Additionally, grounding may help to promote relaxation and reduce stress.

Dental Disorders

Mean: Conditions that affect the teeth and gums.

Grounding: Grounding may help to reduce inflammation and oxidative stress in the teeth and gums in people with dental disorders. Additionally, grounding may help to improve circulation and boost the immune system.

Detached Retina

Mean: A condition in which the retina, the light-sensitive tissue at the back of the eye, separates from the underlying choroid layer.

Grounding: Grounding may help to improve vision and reduce the symptoms of a detached retina by reducing inflammation and oxidative stress in the eyes. Additionally, grounding may help to improve circulation and boost the immune system.

Developmental Delays

Mean: Delays in reaching developmental milestones, such as walking, talking, and social skills.

Grounding: Grounding may help to improve developmental skills and reduce the symptoms of developmental delays by reducing inflammation and oxidative stress in the brain. Additionally, grounding may help to promote relaxation and reduce stress.

Diarrhea

Mean: Loose or watery stool.

Grounding: Grounding may help to improve digestion and reduce diarrhea by reducing inflammation and oxidative stress in the digestive tract. Additionally, grounding may help to promote relaxation and reduce stress.

Digestive problems

Mean: Conditions that affect the digestive system, such as stomach upset, indigestion, and heartburn.

Grounding: Grounding may help to improve digestion and reduce digestive problems by reducing inflammation and oxidative stress in the digestive tract. Additionally, grounding may help to promote relaxation and reduce stress.

Diverticulitis

Mean: Inflammation of small pouches that form in the colon (diverticula).

Grounding: Grounding may help to reduce inflammation and oxidative stress in the colon in people with diverticulitis. Additionally, grounding may help to improve circulation and boost the immune system.

Drug Addiction

Mean: A chronic disease characterized by compulsive drug use and loss of control over drug use.

Grounding: Grounding may help to reduce drug cravings and withdrawal symptoms in people with drug addiction. Additionally, grounding may help to promote relaxation and reduce stress.

Dry Eye Syndrome

Mean: A condition in which the eyes do not produce enough tears, or the tears evaporate too quickly.

Grounding: Grounding may help to reduce inflammation and oxidative stress in the eyes in people with dry eye syndrome. Additionally, grounding may help to improve circulation and boost the immune system.

Ear Infections

Mean: Infections of the ear.

Grounding: Grounding may help to reduce inflammation and oxidative stress in the ears in people with ear infections. Additionally, grounding may help to improve circulation and boost the immune system.

Electro Hypersensitivity

Mean: A condition in which people experience symptoms such as headaches, fatigue, and skin problems in response to exposure to electromagnetic fields.

Grounding: Grounding may help to reduce the symptoms of electro hypersensitivity by reducing inflammation and oxidative stress in the body. Additionally, grounding may help to promote relaxation and reduce stress.

Endometrial Hyperplasia

Mean: A condition in which the lining of the uterus (endometrium) becomes thickened.

Grounding: Grounding may help to reduce inflammation and oxidative stress in the uterus in people with endometrial hyperplasia. Additionally, grounding may help to promote relaxation and reduce stress.

Environmental Allergies

Mean: Allergies to substances in the environment, such as pollen, dust mites, and pet dander.

Grounding: Grounding may help to reduce the symptoms of environmental allergies by reducing inflammation and oxidative stress in the body. Additionally, grounding may help to promote relaxation and reduce stress.

Epilepsy

Mean: A neurological disorder characterized by recurrent seizures.

Grounding: Grounding may help to reduce the frequency and severity of seizures in people with epilepsy. Additionally, grounding may help to promote relaxation and reduce stress.

Eye Floaters

Mean: Small, dark shapes that float around in the field of vision.

Grounding: Grounding may help to improve vision and reduce the visibility of eye floaters by reducing inflammation and oxidative stress in the eyes. Additionally, grounding may help to improve circulation and boost the immune system.

Fatigue

Mean: Extreme tiredness or lack of energy.

Grounding: Grounding may help to improve energy levels and reduce fatigue by reducing inflammation and oxidative stress in the body. Additionally, grounding may help to promote relaxation and improve sleep quality.

Fibroids

Mean: Non-cancerous tumors that grow in the uterus.

Grounding: Grounding may help to reduce the size and symptoms of fibroids by reducing inflammation and oxidative stress in the uterus. Additionally, grounding may help to promote relaxation and reduce stress.

Food Sensitivities

Mean: A condition in which the body has an adverse reaction to certain foods.

Grounding: Grounding may help to reduce inflammation and oxidative stress in the body, which can help to improve the symptoms of food sensitivities. Additionally, grounding may help to promote relaxation and reduce stress.

Gallstones

Mean: Hardened deposits of bile that form in the gallbladder.

Grounding: Grounding may help to reduce inflammation and oxidative stress in the gallbladder, which can help to prevent and reduce the symptoms of gallstones. Additionally, grounding may help to promote relaxation and reduce stress.

Gastritis

Mean: Inflammation of the lining of the stomach.

Grounding: Grounding may help to reduce inflammation and oxidative stress in the stomach, which can help to improve the symptoms of gastritis. Additionally, grounding may help to promote relaxation and reduce stress.

Gastroesophageal Reflux Disease (GERD)

Mean: A condition in which stomach acid backs up (refluxes) into the esophagus.

Grounding: Grounding may help to reduce inflammation and oxidative stress in the esophagus, which can help to improve the symptoms of GERD. Additionally, grounding may help to promote relaxation and reduce stress.

Glaucoma

Mean: A group of eye diseases that damage the optic nerve and can lead to vision loss.

Grounding: Grounding may help to reduce inflammation and oxidative stress in the optic nerve, which can help to prevent and reduce the progression of glaucoma. Additionally, grounding may help to improve circulation and boost the immune system.

Gluten Intolerance

Mean: A condition in which the body is unable to digest gluten, a protein found in wheat, barley, and rye.

Grounding: Grounding may help to reduce inflammation and oxidative stress in the digestive tract in people with gluten intolerance. Additionally, grounding may help to improve circulation and boost the immune system.

Gout

Mean: A type of arthritis that is caused by a buildup of uric acid crystals in the joints.

Grounding: Grounding may help to reduce inflammation and oxidative stress in the joints in people with gout. Additionally, grounding may help to improve circulation and boost the immune system.

Grave's Disease

Mean: An autoimmune disease that causes the thyroid gland to overproduce hormones.

Grounding: Grounding may help to reduce inflammation and oxidative stress in the thyroid gland in people with Grave's disease. Additionally, grounding may help to promote relaxation and reduce stress.

Gum diseases

Mean: Conditions that affect the gums, such as gingivitis and periodontitis.

Grounding: Grounding may help to reduce inflammation and oxidative stress in the gums in people with gum diseases. Additionally, grounding may help to improve circulation and boost the immune system.

Heart Disease

Mean: A group of conditions that affect the heart and blood vessels.

Grounding: Grounding may help to improve cardiovascular health and reduce the risk of heart disease by reducing inflammation and oxidative stress in the heart and blood vessels. Additionally, grounding may help to promote relaxation and reduce stress.

Heartburn

Mean: A burning sensation in the chest that is caused by stomach acid backing up into the esophagus.

Grounding: Grounding may help to reduce inflammation and oxidative stress in the esophagus, which can help to improve heartburn symptoms. Additionally, grounding may help to promote relaxation and reduce stress.

Heavy Metal Toxicity

Mean: A condition in which the body contains high levels of heavy metals, such as lead, mercury, and cadmium.

Grounding: Grounding may help to remove heavy metals from the body and reduce the symptoms of heavy metal toxicity. Additionally, grounding may help to reduce inflammation and oxidative stress.

Hemorrhoids

Mean: Swollen veins in the rectum or anus.

Grounding: Grounding may help to reduce inflammation and oxidative stress in the rectum and anus, which can help to improve the symptoms of hemorrhoids. Additionally, grounding may help to improve circulation and boost the immune system.

Hepatitis

Mean: Inflammation of the liver.

Grounding: Grounding may help to reduce inflammation Herpes Simplex

Herpes Zoster (Shingles)

Mean: A viral infection that causes a rash with blisters and pain, usually on one side of the body.

Grounding: Grounding may help to reduce the frequency and severity of shingles outbreaks by reducing inflammation and oxidative stress in the body. Additionally, grounding may help to promote relaxation and reduce pain.

High blood pressure

Mean: A condition in which the force of blood against the artery walls is too high.

Grounding: Grounding may help to lower blood pressure and improve cardiovascular health by reducing inflammation and oxidative stress in the blood vessels. Additionally, grounding may help to promote relaxation and reduce stress.

High Cholesterol

Mean: A condition in which the levels of cholesterol in the blood are too high.

Grounding: Grounding may help to lower cholesterol levels and improve cardiovascular health by reducing inflammation and oxidative stress in the body. Additionally, grounding may help to promote relaxation and reduce stress.

Hormonal Imbalances

Mean: A condition in which the body produces too much or too little of certain hormones.

Grounding: Grounding may help to balance hormone levels and improve overall health by reducing inflammation and oxidative stress in the body. Additionally, grounding may help to promote relaxation and reduce stress.

Hypothyroidism

Mean: A condition in which the thyroid gland does not produce enough hormones.

Grounding: Grounding may help to improve thyroid function and reduce the symptoms of hypothyroidism by reducing inflammation and oxidative stress in the thyroid gland. Additionally, grounding may help to promote relaxation and reduce stress.

Hypoxia

Mean: A condition in which the body's tissues do not receive enough oxygen.

Grounding: Grounding may help to improve oxygen levels in the blood and reduce the symptoms of hypoxia by improving circulation. Additionally, grounding may help to reduce inflammation and oxidative stress in the body.

Indigestion

Mean: Difficulty digesting food.

Grounding: Grounding may help to improve digestion and reduce indigestion by reducing inflammation and oxidative stress in the digestive tract. Additionally, grounding may help to promote relaxation and reduce stress.

Infertility

Mean: The inability to conceive a child after one year of regular unprotected sexual intercourse.

Grounding: Grounding may help to improve fertility by reducing inflammation and oxidative stress in the body. Additionally, grounding may help to promote relaxation and reduce stress.

Jet lag

Mean: A temporary sleep disorder that can occur after traveling across multiple time zones.

Grounding: Grounding may help to reduce the symptoms of jet lag by resetting the circadian rhythm and improving sleep quality. Additionally, grounding may help to reduce inflammation and oxidative stress, which can also contribute to jet lag symptoms.

Kidney Disorders

Mean: A group of conditions that affect the kidneys.

Grounding: Grounding may help to improve kidney function and reduce the symptoms of kidney disorders by reducing inflammation and oxidative stress in the kidneys. Additionally, grounding may help to improve circulation and boost the immune system.

Kidney Stones

Mean: Hard deposits that form in the kidneys.

Grounding: Grounding may help to prevent and reduce the symptoms of kidney stones by reducing inflammation and oxidative stress in the kidneys. Additionally, grounding may help to improve circulation and boost the immune system.

Lactose Intolerance

Mean: A condition in which the body is unable to digest lactose, a sugar found in milk and other dairy products.

Grounding: Grounding may help to improve digestion and reduce the symptoms of lactose intolerance by reducing inflammation and oxidative stress in the digestive tract. Additionally, grounding may help to promote relaxation and reduce stress.

Learning Disabilities

Mean: A group of disorders that can make it difficult to learn and process information.

Grounding: Grounding may help to improve cognitive function and reduce the symptoms of learning disabilities by reducing inflammation and oxidative stress in the brain. Additionally, grounding may help to promote relaxation and reduce stress.

Liver Disorders

Mean: A group of conditions that affect the liver.

Grounding: Grounding may help to improve liver function and reduce the symptoms of liver disorders by reducing inflammation and oxidative stress in the liver. Additionally, grounding may help to improve circulation and boost the immune system.

Macular Degeneration

Mean: A condition that causes damage to the macula, the central part of the retina.

Grounding: Grounding may help to improve vision and reduce the symptoms of macular degeneration by reducing inflammation and oxidative stress in the eyes. Additionally, grounding may help to improve circulation and boost the immune system.

Malabsorption Syndrome

Mean: A condition in which the body cannot properly absorb nutrients from food.

Grounding: Grounding may help to improve digestion and nutrient absorption in people with malabsorption syndrome by reducing inflammation and oxidative stress in the digestive tract. Additionally, grounding may help to promote relaxation and reduce stress.

Meniere's Disease

Mean: A chronic inner ear disorder that can cause vertigo, tinnitus, and hearing loss.

Grounding: Grounding may help to reduce the frequency and severity of Meniere's disease episodes by reducing inflammation and oxidative stress in the inner ear. Additionally, grounding may help to promote relaxation and reduce stress.

Menopausal Symptoms

Mean: The physical and emotional symptoms that occur during menopause, the transition out of reproductive life.

Grounding: Grounding may help to reduce the severity of menopausal symptoms, such as hot flashes, night sweats, and mood swings, by reducing inflammation and oxidative stress in the body. Additionally, grounding may help to promote relaxation and reduce stress.

Metabolic Acidosis

Mean: A condition in which the body produces too much acid or cannot remove enough acid from the blood.

Grounding: Grounding may help to improve blood pH and reduce the symptoms of metabolic acidosis by reducing inflammation and oxidative stress in the body. Additionally, grounding may help to promote relaxation and reduce stress.

Metabolic Alkalosis

Mean: A condition in which the body produces too much base or cannot remove enough base from the blood.

Grounding: Grounding may help to improve blood pH and reduce the symptoms of metabolic alkalosis by reducing inflammation and oxidative stress in the body. Additionally, grounding may help to promote relaxation and reduce stress.

Metabolic Syndrome

Mean: A group of conditions that increase the risk of heart disease, stroke, and type 2 diabetes.

Grounding: Grounding may help to reduce the risk of metabolic syndrome and its associated complications by reducing inflammation and oxidative stress in the body. Additionally, grounding may help to promote relaxation and reduce stress.

Migraines

Mean: A type of headache that is characterized by severe pain, often on one side of the head, and accompanied by nausea, vomiting, and sensitivity to light and sound.

Grounding: Grounding may help to reduce the frequency and severity of migraines by reducing inflammation and oxidative stress in the brain. Additionally, grounding may help to promote relaxation and reduce stress.

Motion Sickness

Mean: A condition that causes nausea, vomiting, and dizziness during travel.

Grounding: Grounding may help to reduce the symptoms of motion sickness by reducing inflammation and oxidative stress in the brain. Additionally, grounding may help to promote relaxation and reduce stress.

Multiple Chemical Sensitivity

Mean: A condition in which people experience a variety of symptoms, such as headaches, fatigue, and respiratory problems, when exposed to low levels of chemicals.

Grounding: Grounding may help to reduce the symptoms of multiple chemical sensitivity by reducing inflammation and oxidative stress in the body. Additionally, grounding may help to promote relaxation and reduce stress.

Muscle Tension

Mean: Tightness or stiffness in the muscles.

Grounding: Grounding may help to reduce muscle tension and pain by reducing inflammation and oxidative stress in the muscles. Additionally, grounding may help to promote relaxation and reduce stress.

Myofascial Pain Syndrome

Mean: A chronic pain condition that affects the fascia, the connective tissue that surrounds the muscles.

Grounding: Grounding may help to reduce pain and improve function in people with myofascial pain syndrome by reducing inflammation and oxidative stress in the fascia. Additionally, grounding may help to promote relaxation and reduce stress.

Myositis

Mean: Inflammation of the muscles.

Grounding: Grounding may help to reduce inflammation and pain in people with myositis by reducing inflammation and oxidative stress in the muscles. Additionally, grounding may help to promote relaxation and reduce stress.

Nerve Pain

Mean: Pain caused by damage to or irritation of nerves.

Grounding: Grounding may help to reduce nerve pain by reducing inflammation and oxidative stress in the nerves. Additionally, grounding may help to promote relaxation and reduce stress.

Neuralgia

Mean: Pain that occurs along the course of a nerve.

Grounding: Grounding may help to reduce neuralgia pain by reducing inflammation and oxidative stress in the nerves. Additionally, grounding may help to promote relaxation and reduce stress.

Neuritis

Mean: Inflammation of a nerve.

Grounding: Grounding may help to reduce inflammation and pain in people with neuritis by reducing inflammation and oxidative stress in the nerves. Additionally, grounding may help to promote relaxation and reduce stress.

Neuropathy

Mean: A condition that damages the nerves.

Grounding: Grounding may help to reduce the symptoms of neuropathy, such as pain, numbness, and tingling, by reducing inflammation and oxidative stress in the nerves. Additionally, grounding may help to promote relaxation and reduce stress.

Obesity

Mean: A condition in which a person has excess body fat.

Grounding: Grounding may help to promote weight loss and improve overall health in people with obesity by reducing inflammation and oxidative stress in the body. Additionally, grounding may help to promote relaxation and reduce stress.

Osteomalacia (Soft Bones)

Mean: A condition in which the bones are soft and weak.

Grounding: Grounding may help to improve bone health and reduce the risk of osteomalacia by increasing the absorption of calcium and other minerals. Additionally, grounding may help to reduce inflammation and oxidative stress in the bones.

Osteopenia

Mean: Low bone density.

Grounding: Grounding may help to improve bone density and reduce the risk of fractures in people with osteopenia by increasing the absorption of calcium and other minerals. Additionally, grounding may help to reduce inflammation and oxidative stress in the bones.

Osteoporosis

Mean: A condition in which the bones become weak and porous, increasing the risk of fractures.

Grounding: Grounding may help to improve bone density and reduce the risk of fractures in people with osteoporosis by increasing the absorption of calcium and other minerals. Additionally, grounding may help to reduce inflammation and oxidative stress in the bones.

Parkinson's disease

Mean: A neurodegenerative disorder that affects the central nervous system and causes tremors, stiffness, and slowness of movement.

Grounding: Grounding may help to improve symptoms of Parkinson's disease, such as tremors, stiffness, and balance problems, by reducing inflammation and oxidative stress in the brain. Additionally, grounding may help to promote relaxation and reduce stress.

Peripheral Arterial Disease (PAD)

Mean: A condition in which the arteries in the legs and feet become narrowed or blocked, reducing blood flow to these areas.

Grounding: Grounding may help to improve circulation and reduce the risk of complications from PAD, such as leg pain, cramping, and wounds that don't heal, by reducing inflammation and oxidative stress in the blood vessels. Additionally, grounding may help to promote relaxation and reduce stress.

Phantom limb pain

Mean: Pain that is felt in a limb that has been amputated.

Grounding: Grounding may help to reduce phantom limb pain by retraining the brain to recognize the missing limb as still being present. Additionally, grounding may help to promote relaxation and reduce stress.

Plantar fasciitis

Mean: Inflammation of the plantar fascia, a thick band of tissue that runs along the bottom of the foot.

Grounding: Grounding may help to reduce inflammation and pain in people with plantar fasciitis by reducing inflammation and oxidative stress in the plantar fascia. Additionally, grounding may help to promote relaxation and reduce stress.

PMDD (Premenstrual Dysphoric Disorder)

Mean: A severe form of premenstrual syndrome (PMS) that is characterized by severe mood swings, irritability, depression, and anxiety.

Grounding: Grounding may help to reduce the symptoms of PMDD, such as mood swings, irritability, depression, and anxiety, by reducing inflammation and oxidative stress in the body. Additionally, grounding may help to promote relaxation and reduce stress.

PMS (Premenstrual Syndrome)

Mean: A group of physical and emotional symptoms that occur in the days or weeks before a woman's menstrual period.

Grounding: Grounding may help to reduce the symptoms of PMS, such as bloating, cramps, mood swings, and irritability, by reducing inflammation and oxidative stress in the body. Additionally, grounding may help to promote relaxation and reduce stress.

Polyps

Mean: Abnormal growths of tissue that can form on the lining of any organ in the body.

Grounding: Grounding may help to reduce the risk of developing polyps and prevent them from growing into cancer by reducing inflammation and oxidative stress in the body. Additionally, grounding may help to promote relaxation and reduce stress.

Psoriasis

Mean: A chronic skin condition that causes red, scaly patches to form on the skin.

Grounding: Grounding may help to reduce the inflammation and scaling associated with psoriasis by reducing inflammation and oxidative stress in the skin. Additionally, grounding may help to promote relaxation and reduce stress.

Radiation Poisoning

Mean: A condition that occurs when the body is exposed to too much radiation.

Grounding: Grounding may help to reduce the symptoms of radiation poisoning, such as fatigue, nausea, and hair loss, by reducing inflammation and oxidative stress in the body. Additionally, grounding may help to promote relaxation and reduce stress.

Restless Legs Syndrome (RLS)

Mean: A neurological disorder that causes an uncontrollable urge to move the legs, usually in the evening or at night.

Grounding: Grounding may help to reduce the symptoms of RLS, such as the urge to move the legs and difficulty sleeping, by reducing inflammation and oxidative stress in the nervous system. Additionally, grounding may help to promote relaxation and reduce stress.

Rosacea

Mean: A chronic skin condition that causes redness, pimples, and flushing of the face.

Grounding: Grounding may help to reduce the inflammation and redness associated with rosacea by reducing inflammation and oxidative stress in the skin. Additionally, grounding may help to promote relaxation and reduce stress.

Schizophrenia

Mean: A mental health condition that can cause hallucinations, delusions, and disordered thinking.

Grounding: Grounding may help to reduce the symptoms of schizophrenia, such as hallucinations and delusions, by reducing inflammation and oxidative stress in the brain. Additionally, grounding may help to promote relaxation and reduce stress.

Seasonal Allergies

Mean: Allergies to substances that are present in the air, such as pollen, dust mites, and pet dander.

Grounding: Grounding may help to reduce the symptoms of seasonal allergies, such as sneezing, runny nose, and itchy eyes, by reducing inflammation and oxidative stress in the body. Additionally, grounding may help to promote relaxation and reduce stress.

Seizure Disorders

Mean: A group of neurological disorders that cause seizures.

Grounding: Grounding may help to reduce the frequency and severity of seizures in people with seizure disorders by reducing inflammation and oxidative stress in the brain. Additionally, grounding may help to promote relaxation and reduce stress.

Sexual Dysfunction

Mean: A condition in which a person has difficulty with any aspect of sexual function, such as desire, arousal, orgasm, or ejaculation.

Grounding: Grounding may help to improve sexual function by reducing inflammation and oxidative stress in the body and mind. Additionally, grounding may help to promote relaxation and reduce stress.

Shingles

Mean: A viral infection that causes a painful rash with blisters, usually on one side of the body.

Grounding: Grounding may help to reduce the pain and duration of shingles outbreaks by reducing inflammation and oxidative stress in the body. Additionally, grounding may help to promote relaxation and reduce stress.

Sudden Infant Death Syndrome (SIDS)

Mean: The sudden and unexplained death of a seemingly healthy baby under the age of one.

Grounding: Grounding may help to reduce the risk of SIDS by reducing inflammation and oxidative stress in the baby's body. Additionally, grounding may help to promote relaxation and reduce stress in the baby's parents.

Tendinitis

Mean: Inflammation of a tendon, a cord of tissue that connects muscle to bone.

Grounding: Grounding may help to reduce inflammation and pain in people with tendinitis by reducing inflammation and oxidative stress in the tendons. Additionally, grounding may help to promote relaxation and reduce stress.

Type 2 Diabetes

Mean: A chronic condition that affects how the body turns food into energy.

Grounding: Grounding may help to improve blood sugar control and reduce the risk of complications from type 2 diabetes, such as heart disease, stroke, and kidney disease, by reducing inflammation and oxidative stress in the body. Additionally, grounding may help to promote relaxation and reduce stress.

Ulcerative colitis

Mean: A chronic inflammatory bowel disease that causes inflammation and ulcers in the colon.

Grounding: Grounding may help to reduce inflammation and symptoms in people with ulcerative colitis by reducing inflammation and oxidative stress in the colon. Additionally, grounding may help to promote relaxation and reduce stress.

Urinary Tract Infections (UTIs)

Mean: Infections of the urinary tract, which includes the bladder, urethra, and kidneys.

Grounding: Grounding may help to reduce the risk of developing UTIs and prevent them from recurring by reducing inflammation and oxidative stress in the urinary tract. Additionally, grounding may help to promote relaxation and reduce stress.

Venous Insufficiency

Mean: A condition in which the veins in the legs have difficulty returning blood to the heart.

Grounding: Grounding may help to improve circulation and reduce the symptoms of venous insufficiency, such as leg swelling, aching, and cramping, by reducing inflammation and oxidative stress in the blood vessels. Additionally, grounding may help to promote relaxation and reduce stress.

Summary of How Grounding Works

Grounding is a simple and natural way to improve your health and well-being. It is the practice of connecting your body to the Earth, which can help to reduce inflammation, pain, stress, and anxiety.

There are a few different ways to ground yourself. The simplest way is to simply walk barefoot outside on the ground. You can also ground yourself by using a grounding mat or sheet, which is a conductive device that can be connected to the Earth.

To ground yourself using a grounding mat:

1. Find a spot on the ground where you can sit or stand comfortably.
2. Spread out the grounding mat on the ground.
3. Sit or stand on the mat with your bare feet or hands.
4. Relax and enjoy the grounding experience.

You can use a grounding mat for as long as you like. Most people find that grounding for even 20-30 minutes per day can provide benefits.

Safety Considerations

Grounding is generally safe for most people. However, there are a few things to keep in mind:

- If you have a pacemaker or other implanted medical device, talk to your doctor before grounding.
- If you have diabetes or other circulatory problems, be careful not to overdo it when grounding.
- If you are pregnant, avoid grounding for extended periods of time.

professional for a proper diagnosis and guidance on the treatment of specific health conditions.

DEBUNKING MYTHS: CLEARING MISCONCEPTIONS ABOUT GROUNDING

Despite the growing awareness and interest in grounding, it is not immune to skepticism and misinformation. As with any practice that questions the status quo and introduces a different way of doing things, grounding has encountered its fair share of myths. This chapter aims to debunk some common misconceptions about grounding, providing clarity and factual information to help you make informed decisions about incorporating this health-enhancing practice into your lifestyle.

Myth 1: Grounding is Just a New Age Fad

Far from being a fleeting trend of the new age movement, grounding is a practice as old as humanity itself. It represents our primordial connection with the Earth, a bond our ancestors naturally acknowledged and lived out. They walked barefoot, slept on the ground, and cultivated the land with their bare hands, intuitively grounding themselves and enjoying the wellness benefits this connection offered.

The resurgence of interest in grounding today is not a novelty but a reawakening, a return to our roots. Modern science, in its quest to understand the world around us and within us, is validating what our ancestors knew instinctively—our deep connection with the Earth can bring profound health benefits.

Myth 2: There's No Scientific Evidence for Grounding

Contrary to this belief, a growing body of research over the past two decades indicates that grounding can have tangible health benefits. Several studies suggest that grounding can improve sleep quality, reduce pain and inflammation, accelerate wound healing, and bring about several other wellness enhancements.

While it's true that more research is warranted, particularly large-scale, controlled studies, the existing evidence provides a compelling basis for the benefits of grounding. It's a field of study that continues to be explored, and each new piece of research contributes to our understanding of this profound practice.

Myth 3: Grounding is Dangerous Because of Electrical Shocks

The practice of grounding, when carried out correctly, is entirely safe. The risk of electrical shock arises from faulty wiring or equipment—not grounding itself. Grounding products designed for indoor use are typically built with built-in safety resistors. These resistors act as safeguarding mechanisms that prevent any risk of electrical shock, ensuring that you can ground yourself safely while indoors.

Myth 4: You Can't Ground if You Live in a City

While it may seem challenging to connect with the Earth in urban jungles, where natural grounding options like walking barefoot in parks may be limited, grounding is still entirely feasible. Grounding tools such as mats, sheets, and bands offer effective alternatives for city dwellers. These products can be used indoors, allowing you to tap into the Earth's energy from the comfort of your home or workplace.

Myth 5: You Need to Spend Hours Grounding for It to be Effective

You don't need to spend large chunks of your day grounding for it to be beneficial. As with most things in life, grounding works on a gradient—the more you do it, the more you stand to benefit. However, even a few minutes of barefoot walking, a brief lunch break spent in contact with the Earth, or sleeping on a grounding sheet can offer health benefits. The goal is not to clock in hours but to incorporate grounding into your routine in a way that suits your lifestyle.

Demystifying these misconceptions about grounding is key to understanding its true value and potential. Grounding is not a mysterious, esoteric practice reserved for a select few. Instead, it's a natural, accessible, and potent tool that everyone can use to enhance their health and well-being.

In the coming chapters, we will continue to explore grounding's potential, looking at its implications for various aspects of health, from chronic diseases to athletic performance, mental health, and beyond. We will also delve deeper into the scientific research behind grounding, providing a comprehensive overview of this fascinating field.

The journey to understanding and embracing grounding is a journey of reconnection—not just with the Earth, but also with ourselves. By debunking these myths, we clear the path for a more grounded, healthier, and fulfilling life. Grounding is more than a practice—it's a return to our natural state of being, a reclaiming of our ancestral bond with the Earth, and a stepping stone towards holistic well-being.

TESTIMONIAL

1. Personal Experiences with Earthing

As we delve into real-life accounts of earthing experiences, we find a wealth of testimonies that illustrate the profound impact grounding can have on both physical and emotional well-being.

Take for instance James, a construction worker who suffered from chronic back pain for years. It was during a casual conversation with a coworker about alternative healing that he first heard about grounding. Intrigued, he began taking daily barefoot walks in the park and practiced grounding meditation. To his amazement, within weeks, he found significant relief from his chronic pain. The daily regimen of earthing seemed to ease the inflammation, offering him a sense of comfort he had not experienced in years.

Similarly, Maria, a professional tennis player, shared how grounding transformed her athletic performance. Overwhelmed with frequent muscle injuries and slow recovery times, she decided to incorporate grounding into her routine. She invested in a grounding sleep system and earthing shoes, and within a few weeks, she observed a notable difference. Her recovery time improved dramatically, she felt more energetic, and her performance levels surged, leading her to believe in the power of grounding.

Another inspiring testimony comes from Robert, a software engineer dealing with high levels of stress and anxiety due to his demanding work schedule. In his quest for a stress-management strategy, Robert stumbled upon grounding exercises and mindfulness practices. As he began spending his breaks barefoot in the nearby park and practicing grounding mindfulness exercises, he felt his anxieties diminish. The grounding practices seemed to offer him a sense of balance and peace he had never experienced before.

2. The Transformative Power of Grounding

In many instances, grounding practices have brought about transformational changes, instilling renewed health and well-being in practitioners.

Consider Lucy, a woman who struggled with insomnia for decades. After trying countless remedies and therapies, she turned to grounding as a last resort. She purchased a grounding sleep system and also started practicing grounding meditation before bedtime. Gradually, her sleep patterns improved, and before long, she was sleeping soundly through the night for the first time in years. Grounding brought about a transformation in her life that she never thought possible.

John, who had suffered from a chronic inflammatory condition for a long time, shares another powerful testament to grounding's healing potential. His condition often caused him severe discomfort, affecting his quality of life. Intrigued by the potential benefits of grounding, he began spending more time outdoors, barefoot, and engaged in earthing techniques. Over time, he observed a significant reduction in his inflammation and associated pain. John credits grounding as a game-changer in his health journey.

Lastly, the story of Amanda, a young woman who had been grappling with depression and anxiety for years. In her darkest moments, she discovered grounding. She began to spend time outdoors, grounding herself barefoot and practicing grounding exercises. This new routine ignited a sense of connection to the Earth she had never felt before. As she continued her grounding practices, she found emotional balance and a renewed sense of purpose, leading her to label grounding as her pathway to emotional healing.

These personal accounts underscore the transformative power of grounding. They serve as inspiring reminders of the healing potential of the Earth and our inherent need to reconnect with the natural environment. By sharing these stories, we hope to inspire you to explore the benefits of earthing and discover your personal grounding journey.

3. Grounding in the Everyday

Just as grounding can induce remarkable changes, it can also have a profound impact on everyday life, as seen in the experiences of many individuals.

Take for example, Susan, a school teacher who used to feel chronically fatigued. She heard about grounding from a colleague and decided to give it a shot. She began with short barefoot walks in her backyard and used a grounding mat at home. Gradually, she noticed a change in her energy levels. The fatigue that once shadowed her days began to dissipate, and she started feeling more energized and ready to take on her daily tasks.

Similarly, Daniel, a corporate executive, found grounding to be a powerful antidote to work-related stress. His hectic schedule left him feeling drained and stressed. When he learned about grounding, he decided to experiment with grounding techniques during his breaks, going barefoot in the grass around his office building. The results were noticeable. He found himself feeling more relaxed and focused, which significantly improved his productivity and overall work experience.

4. Grounding and Emotional Health

For many individuals, grounding has been a lifeline in their emotional health journey.

Consider the case of Emma, who was dealing with grief after losing a loved one. Amid the emotional turmoil, she discovered grounding. She began spending quiet moments outdoors, barefoot on the grass, feeling the Earth beneath her. Grounding became a therapeutic practice that helped her navigate her grief and restore her emotional balance over time.

Then there's Alex, a military veteran who struggled with post-traumatic stress disorder (PTSD). He discovered grounding through a fellow veteran. As he started practicing regular grounding, combined with therapy, he found his PTSD symptoms significantly decreased. He credits grounding for helping him reconnect with himself and regain his emotional stability.

5. Grounding and Children

The impact of grounding is not limited to adults. Many children have also benefited from grounding practices, as observed by parents and caregivers.

One such case is that of Lily, an eight-year-old diagnosed with attention deficit hyperactivity disorder (ADHD). Her mother introduced grounding as part of Lily's routine, encouraging her to play and walk barefoot outdoors. Remarkably, Lily's attention span increased, and her hyperactivity decreased over time. Her mother firmly believes that grounding played a key role in Lily's improved behavior and cognitive performance.

These accounts, ranging from daily life improvements to emotional healing to benefits in children, highlight the versatile advantages of grounding. They illustrate how grounding, despite its simplicity, has the potential to profoundly impact our health and well-being. By sharing these stories, we hope to encourage you to embrace grounding, reconnect with the Earth, and discover your unique journey towards enhanced health and wellness.

6. Grounding and the Elderly

Grounding is not limited by age, and the elderly community has also reported remarkable experiences.

Take the case of John, a 72-year-old retiree with arthritis. He was struggling with joint pain and stiffness until his granddaughter suggested grounding. Skeptical but willing to try anything, John began spending part of his morning reading the newspaper barefoot in his garden. Over time, he noticed a reduction in his arthritis symptoms. His mobility improved, and he could enjoy his gardening hobby with significantly less discomfort.

In another instance, we have Helen, an 80-year-old, who was dealing with persistent insomnia. Her daughter introduced her to grounding sheets. Despite her initial reservations, Helen found her sleep patterns improved noticeably after starting to use grounding sheets. She began waking up feeling more rested and energized, a feeling she hadn't experienced in years.

7. Grounding and the Workplace

Many professionals have turned to grounding to enhance their work life, finding it improves their health and productivity.

Consider Michael, a software engineer, who started using a grounding mat at his workstation after reading about its benefits. He noticed an increase in his focus and reduction in work-related stress. Michael attributes his enhanced productivity and better work-life balance to his grounding practice.

Similarly, Lisa, a manager at a corporate firm, introduced grounding breaks for her team, encouraging them to walk barefoot in the park next to their office building. She reported a notable increase in team morale, creativity, and overall productivity. The grounding breaks, she believes, added a sense of wellness to their busy corporate life.

8. Grounding and Pets

Grounding benefits are not just for humans; pets can reap these benefits too.

Sarah, a dog owner, observed her pet dog, Max, was more relaxed and had better sleep quality after she started taking him for regular walks in the park, allowing him to walk barefoot on the grass. Max's anxiet around loud noises also seemed to reduce significantly.

In another case, Tom, a cat owner, introduced a grounding mat into his pet's bed. He reported a decrease in his cat's aggressive behavior and an improvement in her overall health.

These stories give us insight into the broad applicability and benefits of grounding. From the elderly to the workplace, even our beloved pets, grounding proves to be a boon. These testimonies serve as real-life evidence that grounding can help improve physical health, enhance emotional well-being, and overall, enrich the quality of life.

9. Grounding in Family Life

Grounding has also found its way into family routines, creating a holistic environment of health and connection.

For example, the Johnson family, who have three young children, started practicing grounding together as a weekend activity. They spend time in their backyard, gardening and playing games, all barefoot. The parents, Laura and Jim, have reported that not only has their family bond strengthened, but their children seem healthier and more calm. Their youngest, who used to frequently fall ill, has had fewer colds since they started this practice.

In another case, the Smith family has made a ritual of grounding picnics. During these picnics, they walk barefoot, play games and enjoy nature. Susan Smith, the mother, reports that these grounding picnics have led to fewer disagreements at home and overall improved the family's mood. She also noticed her seasonal allergies have significantly decreased since they started this practice.

10. Grounding and Mindfulness Practices

Many individuals combine grounding with mindfulness practices, leading to enhanced spiritual and mental health benefits.

Megan, a yoga instructor, introduced grounding mats in her yoga classes. Her students reported an enhanced sense of connection and tranquility during their practice. Megan herself experienced improved energy levels and a deeper sense of balance and grounding.

Likewise, Alex, a mindfulness coach, encourages his clients to practice barefoot meditation outdoors. Alex's clients reported experiencing a deeper connection with themselves and their environment, along with a reduction in stress and anxiety levels. One of his clients, dealing with PTSD, found this practice particularly beneficial in managing their anxiety and improving their mental health.

Grounding, when integrated into our lives, becomes more than just a health practice. It connects us back to nature, enhances our relationships, and complements our spiritual practices. These real-life stories reaffirm the multitude of benefits that grounding brings into our lives, pushing us toward an improved sense of health, well-being, and connection with the world around us.

11. Grounding and Sports Performance

Grounding has also become popular among athletes for its perceived benefits in recovery and performance.

Peter, a marathon runner, started incorporating grounding practices into his post-workout routine. He would cool down by walking barefoot on the grass. To his surprise, he started to notice faster recovery times and fewer injuries, leading to improved training sessions and better performance in his races.

Similarly, Angela, a professional tennis player, was introduced to grounding shoes by her coach. She noticed that her endurance seemed to increase and that she felt more energized during her games. The usual discomfort she used to feel in her knees also lessened, which she attributes to her new grounding practices.

12. Grounding in the Workplace

In the face of rising work-related stress and the need for work-life balance, some companies and employees have started to explore grounding as a part of workplace wellness initiatives.

Mike, an HR manager at a tech company, introduced grounding mats in breakout spaces within the office. He also organized 'Grounding Fridays', encouraging employees to spend lunch breaks barefoot in the nearby park. Employees reported reduced stress levels, increased focus, and improved work-life balance, which they associated with these grounding practices.

Rachel, a freelance graphic designer, turned to grounding to help manage the loneliness and anxiety that came with working from home. She started her day with a barefoot walk in her garden, took regular grounding breaks, and used a grounding mat under her desk. She found that grounding not only helped alleviate her anxiety but also boosted her creativity and productivity.

These stories from athletes and working professionals highlight the potential of grounding to improve physical performance, mental clarity, and workplace well-being.

13. Grounding and Elderly Health

Grounding has shown promise in addressing some of the common health concerns among the elderly population.

Eleanor, an 82-year-old woman, suffered from chronic arthritis and insomnia. Her daughter introduced her to grounding, starting with a grounding mat for her bed and short barefoot walks in the park. Within weeks, Eleanor reported an improvement in her sleep and a reduction in her pain levels.

Similarly, George, a 75-year-old retired teacher, used to feel constantly fatigued and had high blood pressure. He started spending an hour every afternoon sitting barefoot in his garden, reading. Over a few months, he noticed increased energy levels and improved mood. His blood pressure also started to stabilize.

These examples show the positive effects grounding can have on the overall well-being and quality of life of the elderly, indicating that it's never too late to start this practice.

14. Grounding and Children's Development

With increasing screen time and decreasing outdoor play, grounding can play a vital role in children's physical and emotional development.

Jessica, a school teacher, started incorporating grounding activities in her kindergarten class. She introduced 'barefoot playtimes' and 'outdoor learning sessions', where children would engage with the earth directly. Not only did she notice improvements in children's attention span, but parents also reported better sleep patterns and reduced hyperactivity at home.

Similarly, Olivia, a mother of two, established a 'family grounding time' every evening where they would walk barefoot in their backyard or play games on the grass. She saw a significant difference in her children's stress levels and overall mood, making their family time more enjoyable and bonding.

15. Grounding and Pet Health

Pets, just like humans, can potentially benefit from grounding.

Sarah, a pet owner, noticed that her indoor cat seemed anxious and suffered from frequent infections. She started allowing her cat outside for a few hours each day to roam in the yard. Over time, the cat's anxiety reduced, and her health improved. Sarah is convinced that the grounding effect of direct contact with the Earth benefited her pet's overall well-being.

In another instance, Martin, a vet, recommended a client with a dog recovering from surgery to let the dog lie on a grounding mat. The dog's owner was pleasantly surprised by the speedy recovery and the dog's increased energy levels post-surgery.

By sharing these testimonials from various walks of life - from athletes to the elderly, from children to pets - this section underscores the widespread applicability and potential benefits of grounding. These stories serve to inspire readers to explore and embrace grounding in their routines, offering a promise of a healthier, more balanced life.

FREQUENTLY ASK QUESTIONS

What is grounding/earthing? Grounding, also known as earthing, is a practice that involves direct physical contact with the surface of the Earth, such as walking barefoot on grass or soil. It is based on the principle that the Earth's surface possesses a limitless supply of free electrons that can neutralize harmful free radicals in our bodies.

How does grounding work scientifically? Grounding works on the principle of electrical conductivity. The Earth maintains a negative electrical potential, and when we make direct contact with the Earth's surface, our bodies can absorb these negative electrons. This can neutralize free radicals and reduce inflammation, among other health benefits.

What are the potential benefits of grounding? Potential benefits of grounding include reduction of inflammation, stress relief, improved sleep quality, faster healing of injuries, improved cardiovascular health, enhanced immune function, increased energy, and improved mood.

Is there any scientific evidence supporting the practice of grounding? Yes, numerous scientific studies and research articles have reported the benefits of grounding. These studies have shown that grounding can improve sleep, reduce inflammation, and promote overall health. However, more comprehensive research is still needed to fully understand all its potential benefits.

How often should I practice grounding to experience its benefits? While there's no hard and fast rule, experts suggest that you should aim for at least 30 minutes to an hour of grounding each day to experience its benefits. However, even a few minutes can be beneficial.

Can grounding help reduce stress and anxiety? Yes, grounding has been shown to help reduce stress and anxiety by normalizing cortisol (the stress hormone) levels and promoting a state of relaxation.

How can grounding improve my sleep? Grounding can improve sleep by normalizing the day-night cortisol rhythm, which promotes better sleep quality and duration.

Can grounding aid in pain management? Yes, grounding may help alleviate chronic pain. This is believed to be due to its ability to reduce inflammation, which is often a cause of chronic pain.

Is grounding beneficial for cardiovascular health? Some studies have indicated that grounding may improve cardiovascular health by reducing blood viscosity and improving circulation, though more research is needed.

Can grounding help with inflammation and immunity? Yes, grounding can help reduce inflammation and boost immunity. By absorbing negative electrons from the Earth, grounding can neutralize free radicals and reduce oxidative stress, which supports a healthy immune system.

What are some common grounding techniques? Common grounding techniques include walking barefoot on the earth, swimming in natural bodies of water, gardening with bare hands, or using grounding products such as grounding mats or sheets.

Can I practice grounding indoors? Yes, there are grounding products available, like grounding mats, sheets, and bands that can be used indoors. These products are connected to the Earth via a wire and a grounded wall outlet.

What grounding products are available for indoor use? A variety of grounding products are available for indoor use, including grounding mats, sheets, patches, bands, and even grounding shoes. These products are designed to help you experience the benefits of grounding when direct contact with the Earth isn't possible.

Is it safe to use grounding products during a thunderstorm? While grounding products are generally safe, it's advised to disconnect them during a thunderstorm as a precautionary measure.

Are there any side effects or risks of grounding? Grounding is generally considered safe. However, individuals with certain conditions, like those on blood thinners, should consult their healthcare provider before beginning grounding practices, as grounding can thin the blood slightly.

DICTIONARY

1. **ACNE**: Acne is a skin condition that can cause pimples and blackheads, especially in teenagers.
2. **ACOUSTIC THERAPY**: Acoustic therapy is a treatment that uses sound or music to help people relax or feel better.
3. **ACUITY**: Acuity means having sharpness or keenness, like having good vision to see small details.
4. **ACUPUNCTURE**: Acupuncture is a type of therapy where tiny needles are inserted into your skin to help with pain or other health issues.
5. **ADRENAL IMBALANCE**: Adrenal imbalance means that the glands near your kidneys, called the adrenal glands, are not working properly.
6. **ADVANTAGEOUS**: Advantageous means something that is helpful or beneficial in some way.
7. **ADVOCACY**: Advocacy is when you speak up for or support a particular cause or idea.
8. **ALTRUISM**: Altruism is when people do things to help others, even if they don't get anything in return.
9. **AMALGAM**: An amalgam is a mixture or blend of different things, like a mix of metals.
10. **AMALGAMATION**: Amalgamation is the process of mixing or combining different things to make one.
11. **AMETHYST**: Amethyst is a purple gemstone that is often used in jewelry.

12. **ANECDOTAL**: Anecdotal means something based on personal stories or experiences rather than scientific evidence.

13. **ANECDOTAL**: Anecdotal is the same as before, it means something based on personal stories or experiences rather than scientific evidence.

14. **ANECDOTALLY**: Anecdotally is the adverb form of anecdotal, used to describe something done based on personal stories or experiences.

15. **ANTI-INFLAMMATORY**: Anti-inflammatory means something that helps reduce swelling and pain, often used for medicines.

16. **ANTIOXIDANTS**: Antioxidants are substances that help protect your body from damage caused by harmful molecules called free radicals.

17. **ANXIETY**: Anxiety is a feeling of worry or fear, often about something that might happen in the future.

18. **ANXIOUS STATES**: Anxious states are times when someone is feeling nervous or worried.

19. **APPLICABLE**: Applicable means that something is relevant or can be used in a particular situation.

20. **ARGUABLY**: Arguably means something that can be debated or discussed, often because it's not clear-cut.

21. **ARTHRITIS**: Arthritis is a medical condition where the joints in your body can be painful and swollen.

22. **ARTISTIC**: Artistic means having to do with art or being creative.

23. **ARTISTIC EXPRESSION**: Artistic expression is a way to show your creativity or feelings through art, like painting or music.

24. **ATTENTION DEFICIT HYPERACTIVITY DISORDER (ADHD)**: ADHD is a condition where it's hard to focus and sit still, and you might be very active and impulsive.

25. **AUGMENTED**: Augmented means something that is made bigger or enhanced in some way.

26. **AUGMENTING HEALING**: Augmenting healing means making the process of getting better or healing stronger or more effective.

27. **AUTOIMMUNE DISEASES**: Autoimmune diseases are conditions where your immune system mistakenly attacks your own body.

28. **AUTONOMIC NERVOUS SYSTEM (ANS)**: The autonomic nervous system is a part of your body that controls things like your heartbeat and digestion without you having to think about it.

29. **AYURVEDA**: Ayurveda is a traditional system of medicine from India that focuses on balancing the body and mind.

30. **BALM**: A balm is a soothing substance, often used for healing or moisturizing the skin.

31. **BAREFOOT CARDIO**: Barefoot cardio means doing exercises like running or jumping without wearing shoes.

32. **BIOCHEMICAL PROCESSES**: Biochemical processes are chemical reactions that happen inside living organisms, like how your body breaks down food.

33. **BIODIVERSITY**: Biodiversity is the variety of different plants and animals in a particular ecosystem.

34. **BIOELECTRIC MILIEU**: The bioelectric milieu refers to the electrical activity happening within a living organism.

35. **BIOLOGICAL**: Biological means relating to living things or organisms.

36. **BOLSTER IMMUNE**: Bolster immune means to strengthen or support the body's immune system, which helps fight off sickness.

37. **BOLSTERING**: Bolstering means strengthening or improving something.

38. **BOOST IMMUNE HEALTH**: Boosting immune health means doing things to make your immune system stronger and better at protecting you from illnesses.

39. **BOOSTED PARASYMPATHETIC ACTIVITY**: Boosted parasympathetic activity means increasing the part of your nervous system that helps you relax and rest.

40. **BOOSTING VITALITY**: Boosting vitality means increasing your energy and liveliness.

41. **BRAIN HEALTH**: Brain health means taking care of your brain and keeping it working well.

42. **BURGEONING**: Burgeoning means something that is growing or developing rapidly.

43. **CARDIOVASCULAR**: Cardiovascular refers to the heart and blood vessels in your body.

44. **CATALYST**: A catalyst is something that makes a chemical reaction happen faster.

45. **CAVEATS**: Caveats are warnings or conditions that you should be aware of before doing something.

46. **CELL**: A cell is the basic unit of life, like a tiny building block that makes up living things.

47. **CELLULAR**: Cellular means related to or involving cells.

48. **CHAMOMILE**: Chamomile is a type of flower often used to make calming tea.

49. **CHRONIC ARTHRITIS**: Chronic arthritis is a long-lasting condition where your joints can be painful and swollen.

50. **CHRONIC CONDITIONS**: Chronic conditions are health problems that last a long time or keep coming back.

51. **CHRONIC INFLAMMATION**: Chronic inflammation is long-lasting swelling in your body.

52. **CHRONIC PAIN**: Chronic pain is ongoing and persistent discomfort or soreness.

53. **CHRONIC STRESS**: Chronic stress is long-term worry or tension that can affect your health.

54. **CIRCADIAN**: Circadian refers to the natural rhythm or cycle that your body goes through in a day, like waking and sleeping.

55. **CIRCADIAN RHYTHMS**: Circadian rhythms are the regular patterns of changes in your body that happen over a 24-hour period.

56. **CLEAR QUARTZ**: Clear quartz is a type of crystal that is transparent and often used in jewelry or decorations.

57. **COALESCE**: Coalesce means coming together or merging into one.

58. **COGNITIVE**: Cognitive relates to thinking, learning, and understanding.

59. **COGNITIVE HARMONY**: Cognitive harmony means having a balance in your thinking and mental processes.

60. **COGNITIVE PROCESSES**: Cognitive processes are the ways your brain works to think, learn, and remember

61. **COGNITIVE SHARPNESS**: Cognitive sharpness means having a clear and alert mind, being able to think quickly.

62. **COGNITIVE SYMBIOSIS**: Cognitive symbiosis refers to a balanced and mutually beneficial relationship between different mental processes.

63. **COHESION**: Cohesion is the act of sticking together or being united as a group.

64. **COMMUNION**: Communion means a close connection or sharing of thoughts and feelings with others.

65. **COMPLEMENTARY THERAPIES**: Complementary therapies are alternative treatments used alongside traditional medicine to promote healing and well-being.

66. **CONVERGENCE**: Convergence is the process of different things coming together or meeting at a common point.

67. **CORONARY ARTERY DISEASE**: Coronary artery disease is a condition where the blood vessels supplying the heart become narrow or blocked.

68. **CORTISOL**: Cortisol is a hormone produced by the body in response to stress.

69. **CORTISOL CONTROL**: Cortisol control refers to managing the levels of cortisol in the body to reduce stress.

70. **CORTISOL LEVELS**: Cortisol levels are the amounts of cortisol present in the bloodstream.

71. **CORTISOL REGULATION**: Cortisol regulation means controlling and maintaining the proper levels of cortisol in the body.

72. **CROSS-POLLINATION**: Cross-pollination is the transfer of pollen from one flower to another, promoting plant reproduction.

73. **CRYSTALS**: Crystals are solid substances with a regular geometric shape, often valued for their beauty and energy properties.

74. **DECODING MINDFULNESS**: Decoding mindfulness means understanding and applying the practice of mindfulness, which involves being fully present in the moment.

75. **DECREASING INFLAMMATION**: Decreasing inflammation means reducing the swelling and redness that can occur in the body as a response to injury or illness.

76. **DEFORESTATION**: Deforestation is the process of cutting down and removing forests, often for agricultural or industrial purposes.

77. **DEMEANOR**: Demeanor refers to a person's behavior or outward manner, often reflecting their attitude.

78. **DEPRESSION**: Depression is a mental health condition characterized by persistent feelings of sadness and hopelessness.

79. **DERMATOLOGICAL**: Dermatological relates to the study and treatment of skin-related issues.

80. **DEW-KISSED GRASS**: Dew-kissed grass is grass that is wet with dewdrops from the morning or evening moisture.

81. **DIABETES**: Diabetes is a medical condition where the body has difficulty regulating blood sugar levels.

82. **DIVERSE MICROBIOME**: Diverse microbiome refers to the variety of microorganisms living in a particular environment, like the gut.

83. **DOSHAS**: Doshas are elements in Ayurvedic medicine that represent different body types and energies.

84. **DRY SKIN**: Dry skin is when the skin lacks moisture and can feel rough or flaky.

85. **ECO-CONSCIOUS BEHAVIOR**: Eco-conscious behavior involves making choices that are mindful of the environment and sustainable.

86. **ECOLOGICAL**: Ecological relates to the study of ecosystems and the interactions between organisms and their environments.

87. **ECOSYSTEMS**: Ecosystems are communities of living organisms and their interactions with each other and their physical surroundings.

88. **ECZEMA**: Eczema is a skin condition characterized by itchy and inflamed patches of skin.

89. **EFFICACY**: Efficacy refers to the effectiveness or ability of something to produce desired results.

90. **ELECTRICAL ENERGY**: Electrical energy is the energy produced by the movement of electrons, often used to power devices.

91. **ELECTRICAL IONS**: Electrical ions are charged particles, either positively or negatively charged.

92. **EMOTIONAL EQUANIMITY**: Emotional equanimity means maintaining a calm and balanced emotional state.

93. **EMOTIONAL EQUILIBRIUM**: Emotional equilibrium refers to a stable and balanced emotional state.

94. **EMOTIONAL FREEDOM TECHNIQUES (EFT)**: Emotional Freedom Techniques are practices that aim to release emotional stress and promote well-being.

95. **EMOTIONAL STATES**: Emotional states are different moods and feelings that a person can experience.

96. **EMOTIONAL TURMOIL**: Emotional turmoil is a state of inner turmoil or emotional upheaval.

97. **EMPATHETIC**: Empathetic means being able to understand and share the feelings of others.

98. **EMPIRICAL VALIDATION**: Empirical validation means confirming something through observation and evidence-based research.

99. **ENCAPSULATES**: Encapsulates means to enclose or contain something within a capsule or barrier.

100. **ENDOCRINE SYSTEM**: The endocrine system is a network of glands that produce hormones to regulate various bodily functions.

101. **ENERGETICS**: Energetics refers to the study of energy and its transformations in living organisms.

102. **ENERGY EQUILIBRIUM**: Energy equilibrium is a balanced state of energy within the body.

103. **EQUANIMITY**: Equanimity is a state of calmness and composure, especially in difficult situations.

104. **EQUILIBRIUM**: Equilibrium is a state of balance or stability.

105. **ESOTERIC**: Esoteric refers to knowledge or practices that are understood by only a select few, often considered mysterious or hidden.

106. **EXACERBATES**: Exacerbates means to make a problem or situation worse.

107. **EXISTENTIAL**: Existential relates to questions and concepts about the meaning of life and existence.

108. **FOREST BATHING**: Forest bathing involves immersing oneself in a natural forest environment to promote relaxation and well-being.

109. **FREE ELECTRONS**: Free electrons are electrons that are not bound to atoms and can move freely, often associated with electrical conductivity.

110. **FREE RADICALS**: Free radicals are unstable molecules that can cause damage to cells and tissues.

111. **FRENETIC**: Frenetic means frantic or chaotic, often describing fast and uncontrolled activity.

112. **FRENETIC PACE**: Frenetic pace refers to a very fast and hectic speed or rhythm.

113. **FULCRUM**: A fulcrum is the point on which a lever pivots or balances.

114. **GASTROESOPHAGEAL REFLUX DISEASE (GERD)**: GERD is a condition where stomach acid flows back into the esophagus, causing discomfort.

115. **GINSENG**: Ginseng is a medicinal herb believed to have various health benefits.

116. **GROUNDING AUGMENTS EMOTIONAL AWARENESS**: Grounding, in this context, means connecting with the earth or being emotionally stable, which can enhance one's awareness of emotions.

117. **GUT HEALTH**: Gut health refers to the well-being of the digestive system and its microorganisms.

118. **GUT MICROBIOME**: The gut microbiome is the community of microorganisms living in the digestive tract.

119. **GUT MICROBIOME DIVERSITY**: Gut microbiome diversity is the variety of different

120. **GUT-BRAIN AXIS**: The gut-brain axis is a communication system between the gut and the brain, influencing both physical and mental health.

121. **HARBORING**: Harboring means sheltering or providing a place for something to exist.

122. **HARMONIOUS**: Harmonious means being in agreement or having a pleasant and balanced relationship.

123. **HEALING TOUCH**: Healing touch refers to a therapeutic approach involving gentle physical contact to promote relaxation and well-being.

124. **HEART DISEASE**: Heart disease is a group of conditions that affect the heart's function and can be harmful to health.

125. **HEART FAILURE**: Heart failure is a condition where the heart cannot pump blood effectively, leading to various symptoms.

126. **HEART RATE VARIABILITY**: Heart rate variability is the variation in time between consecutive heartbeats and can be an indicator of overall health.

127. **HOLOTROPIC BREATHWORK**: Holotropic breathwork is a therapeutic technique that involves controlled breathing to induce altered states of consciousness.

128. **HORMONAL EQUILIBRIUM**: Hormonal equilibrium is a balanced state of hormone levels in the body.

129. **HORMONAL HARMONY**: Hormonal harmony means having a state of balance and proper functioning of hormones.

130. **HORMONAL HEALTH**: Hormonal health refers to the overall well-being of the body's hormone systems.

131. **HYPOTHESIS**: A hypothesis is a proposed explanation for a phenomenon, often used as a starting point for scientific investigation.

132. **HYPOTHESIZED**: Hypothesized means to suggest or propose a hypothesis as a possible explanation.

133. **HYPOTHETICAL SYNERGIES**: Hypothetical synergies refer to potential beneficial interactions or cooperation between different elements, often in a theoretical context.

134. **IMMUNE IRREGULARITIES**: Immune irregularities are abnormalities or disruptions in the functioning of the immune system.

135. **IMMUNE SYSTEM**: The immune system is the body's defense mechanism against infections and diseases.

136. **IMMUNE SYSTEM MODULATION**: Immune system modulation refers to the control or adjustment of the immune response.

137. **IMMUNODEFICIENCIES**: Immunodeficiencies are conditions where the immune system is weakened and less effective in protecting the body.

138. **IMMUTABLE**: Immutable means unchangeable or not subject to change.

139. **INESCAPABLE**: Inescapable means impossible to avoid or get away from.

140. **INEXORABLY**: Inexorably means in a manner that is impossible to stop or prevent.

141. **INFLAMMATION**: Inflammation is the body's response to injury or infection, often characterized by redness and swelling.

142. **INFLAMMATORY BOWEL DISEASES (IBD)**: IBD includes conditions like Crohn's disease and ulcerative colitis, which cause chronic inflammation in the digestive tract.

143. **INSOMNIA**: Insomnia is a sleep disorder where people have difficulty falling asleep or staying asleep.

144. **INTRINSIC ENERGIES**: Intrinsic energies refer to the inherent or natural sources of energy within an organism.

145. **INTRINSICALLY**: Intrinsically means inherently or as a fundamental part of something.

146. **INVIGORATE**: Invigorate means to give energy and vitality to something or someone.

147. **INVIGORATING**: Invigorating means making something more lively, energizing, or refreshing.

148. **IRRITABLE BOWEL SYNDROME (IBS)**: IBS is a digestive disorder that can cause symptoms like abdominal pain and changes in bowel habits.

149. **KAPHA**: Kapha is one of the three doshas in Ayurvedic medicine, representing elements of earth and water.

150. **LABYRINTH**: A labyrinth is a complex and winding maze or a design often used for meditation or spiritual purposes.

151. **LAPIS LAZULI**: Lapis lazuli is a blue gemstone prized for its beauty and used in jewelry and art.

152. **LAVENDER**: Lavender is a fragrant purple flower often used for its soothing scent in aromatherapy and beauty products.

153. **LINCHPIN**: A linchpin is a crucial element or person that holds something together.

154. **MACA ROOT**: Maca root is a plant native to Peru, known for its potential health benefits and use as a dietary supplement.

155. **MALAISE**: Malaise is a general feeling of discomfort or uneasiness, often indicating an underlying illness.

156. **MAX'S ANXIETY**: Max's anxiety refers to anxiety experienced by someone named Max, which is a common emotion of worry or unease.

157. **MEDICINAL**: Medicinal relates to the use of substances or treatments for their healing properties.

158. **MEDITATION (DHYANA)**: Meditation, specifically dhyana, is a practice of focusing the mind and achieving a state of deep concentration or relaxation.

159. **MELATONIN REGULATION**: Melatonin regulation refers to the control and balance of melatonin, a hormone that regulates sleep-wake cycles.

160. **MENTAL CLARITY**: Mental clarity means having a clear and focused mind with no confusion.

161. **MENTAL ILLNESSES**: Mental illnesses are conditions that affect a person's emotional and psychological well-being.

162. **MENTAL LUCIDITY**: Mental lucidity means having a clear and sharp mental state with a high level of awareness.

163. **MERIDIANS**: Meridians are energy pathways in traditional Chinese medicine through which vital energy flows.

164. **METABOLIC FUNCTION**: Metabolic function refers to the chemical processes that occur within the body to maintain life.

165. **METABOLIC RATE**: Metabolic rate is the rate at which the body burns calories and processes energy.

166. **METAPHORICAL STANCE**: Metaphorical stance refers to the use of figurative language or symbols to convey a message or perspective.

167. **METAPHYSICAL REALMS**: Metaphysical realms are conceptual or spiritual dimensions beyond the physical world.

168. **METHODOLOGY**: Methodology is the system of methods and principles used in a particular field of study or research.

169. **MICROBES**: Microbes are tiny microorganisms, such as bacteria and viruses, that are often invisible to the naked eye.

170. **MICROBIOME**: The microbiome is the collection of microorganisms living in a particular environment, like the human gut.

171. **MICROORGANISMS**: Microorganisms are tiny living beings, including bacteria, viruses, and fungi.

172. **MINDFUL BREATHING (PRANAYAMA)**: Mindful breathing, or pranayama, is a practice of conscious and controlled breathing often used in yoga and meditation.

173. **MITIGATING**: Mitigating means reducing or lessening the severity of something, such as a problem or risk.

174. **MODALITIES**: Modalities are different methods or approaches used for a particular purpose, often in healthcare or therapy.

175. **MODALITY**: Modality is a singular form of modalities, referring to a specific method or approach.

176. **MODULATE HORMONE LEVELS**: Modulate hormone levels means to adjust or regulate the amounts of hormones in the body.

177. **MODULATE IMMUNE REACTIONS**: Modulate immune reactions means to control or influence how the immune system responds to various stimuli.

178. **MOLECULAR**: Molecular means related to the smallest units of substances, called molecules, that make up matter.

179. **MOLLIFY STRESS**: Mollify stress means to soothe or alleviate feelings of stress and tension.

180. **MOOD DISORDERS**: Mood disorders are conditions that affect a person's emotional state, such as depression or bipolar disorder.

181. **MOOD FLUCTUATIONS**: Mood fluctuations are changes in a person's emotional state that can vary over time.

182. **MULTIDIMENSIONAL**: Multidimensional means having many different aspects or dimensions.

183. **MULTILAYERED**: Multilayered means having multiple layers or levels.

184. **MYRIAD**: Myriad means a countless or immense number of things.

185. **NASCENT STAGES**: Nascent stages are the early or beginning phases of something.

186. **NATURAL ELECTRICAL CHARGE**: Natural electrical charge refers to the inherent electrical properties of certain materials or substances.

187. **NATURAL TERRAINS**: Natural terrains are the landscapes or geographical features of the Earth's surface that haven't been significantly altered by human activities.

188. **NERVOUS SYSTEM**: The nervous system is the body's network of nerves and cells that transmit signals and control various functions.

189. **NEUROLOGICAL CONDITIONS**: Neurological conditions are disorders that affect the nervous system, including the brain and spinal cord.

190. **NEUTRALIZE FREE RADICALS**: Neutralize free radicals means to counteract or eliminate harmful molecules in the body that can cause damage.

191. **NEW WORD LIST**: New word list refers to a collection of words or terms, often organized for specific purposes.

192. **NUANCED**: Nuanced means having subtle differences or variations in meaning or understanding.

193. **NUTRIENT CONVERSION**: Nutrient conversion is the process of changing nutrients from one form to another for use in the body.

194. **NUTRIENT-DENSE DIET**: Nutrient-dense diet means eating foods that are rich in essential nutrients relative to their calorie content.

195. **ODYSSEY**: An odyssey is a long and adventurous journey, often with various challenges and experiences.

196. **OMEGA-3 FATTY ACIDS**: Omega-3 fatty acids are essential fats that are important for good health, often found in certain foods like fish.

197. **ORGANS**: Organs are specialized structures in the body that perform specific functions, such as the heart and lungs.

198. **OVERARCHING**: Overarching means including or encompassing everything, often describing a broad concept or idea.

199. **OXIDATIVE STRESS**: Oxidative stress is an imbalance between the production of harmful free radicals and the body's ability to counteract them. ("Nitric Oxide and Its Crucial Impact on Cardiovascular Health")

200. **PARADIGM-SHIFTING**: Paradigm-shifting refers to a significant change in the way something is understood or approached.

201. **PARASYMPATHETIC NERVOUS SYSTEM (PNS)**: The parasympathetic nervous system is a part of the autonomic nervous system that promotes relaxation and rest.

202. **PATHOGENS**: Pathogens are microorganisms or agents that can cause disease or infection in the body.

203. **PEER-REVIEWED SCIENTIFIC STUDIES**: Peer-reviewed scientific studies are research papers that have been evaluated and approved by experts in the field before publication.

204. **PHOBIAS**: Phobias are extreme and irrational fears of specific objects or situations.

205. **PHYSICAL**: Physical refers to the body and the tangible aspects of the world.

206. **PHYSIOLOGICAL**: Physiological means relating to the normal functions and processes of the body.

207. **PHYSIOLOGICAL FUNCTIONS**: Physiological functions are the natural processes and activities that occur within the body.

208. **PHYSIOLOGICAL PROCESSES**: Physiological processes are the series of actions and changes that take place within living organisms.

209. **PHYSIOLOGICAL RELAXATION**: Physiological relaxation is the state of calmness and ease that affects the body's functions.

210. **PHYSIOLOGY**: Physiology is the study of how living organisms function and operate.

211. **PITTA**: Pitta is one of the three doshas in Ayurvedic medicine, representing elements of fire and water.

212. **PIVOTAL**: Pivotal means being of crucial importance or serving as a central point.

213. **PLETHORA**: Plethora means an excessive or overwhelming amount of something.

214. **POIGNANT**: Poignant means evoking a strong sense of emotion or empathy.

215. **POOR SLEEP QUALITY**: Poor sleep quality refers to sleep that is not restful or refreshing, often due to disruptions or discomfort.

216. **POSES (ASANAS)**: Poses, also known as asanas, are specific body positions and postures used in yoga practice.

217. **POST-TRAUMATIC STRESS DISORDER (PTSD)**: PTSD is a mental health condition that can develop after experiencing a traumatic event.

218. **PREDECESSORS**: Predecessors are people or things that came before and are replaced by others.

219. **PRE-EXISTING HORMONAL CONDITIONS**: Pre-existing hormonal conditions are hormonal imbalances that existed before a specific time or event.

220. **PROPAGATED**: Propagated means spread or transmitted, often referring to information or ideas.

221. **PSORIASIS**: Psoriasis is a skin condition that causes red, scaly patches on the skin.

222. **PSYCHOLOGICAL**: Psychological relates to the mind and mental processes.

223. **PTSD**: PTSD is the abbreviation for post-traumatic stress disorder, a mental health condition resulting from trauma.

224. **QI GONG**: Qi Gong is a Chinese practice involving movement, breathing, and meditation to cultivate and balance life energy.

225. **QUELL INFLAMMATION**: Quell inflammation means to calm or suppress inflammation in the body.

226. **QUELLING**: Quelling means calming, suppressing, or reducing something, often used in the context of emotions or issues.

227. **RADICALS**: Radicals are atoms or molecules with unpaired electrons, often highly reactive.

228. **RAPIDITY**: Rapidity means a high rate of speed or quickness.

229. **REGENERATION**: Regeneration means the process of renewal, growth, or restoration.

230. **REIKI**: Reiki is a healing technique that involves the transfer of energy through touch or non-contact methods.

231. **REJUVENATION**: Rejuvenation means the process of becoming young or revitalized.

232. **REKINDLE**: Rekindle means to revive or renew something, often a feeling or relationship.

233. **RESONATES**: Resonates means to produce a strong and harmonious response or connection.

234. **RESPIRATORY HEALTH**: Respiratory health refers to the well-being of the respiratory system, including the lungs and airways.

235. **ROOT CHAKRA**: The root chakra is the first energy center in the body, located at the base of the spine, and associated with feelings of security and stability.

236. **SACRAL CHAKRA**: The sacral chakra is the second energy center in the body, located in the lower abdomen, and associated with emotions, creativity, and relationships.

237. **SAGE**: Sage is a fragrant herb often used in cooking and smudging rituals for its cleansing properties.

238. **SELF-HEALING**: Self-healing is the practice of using one's own resources and techniques to promote physical or emotional well-being.

239. **SENSES**: Senses are the faculties or abilities through which we perceive the world, including sight, hearing, taste, smell, and touch.

240. **SENSORY PERCEPTION**: Sensory perception is the process of receiving and interpreting information through the senses.

241. **SENSORY STIMULATION**: Sensory stimulation involves activating or exciting the senses, often for therapeutic purposes.

242. **SEROTONIN**: Serotonin is a neurotransmitter in the brain that plays a role in mood regulation and feelings of well-being.

243. **SHAMANIC PRACTICES**: Shamanic practices are spiritual and healing rituals performed by shamans in various cultures.

244. **SLEEP CYCLES**: Sleep cycles are the patterns of alternating sleep stages, including REM (rapid eye movement) and non-REM stages, during a night's sleep.

245. **SLEEP DISORDERS**: Sleep disorders are conditions that disrupt normal sleep patterns and can affect a person's overall health.

246. **SOOTHING AROMAS**: Soothing aromas are fragrances that have a calming or comforting effect on the senses.

247. **SOOTHING MUSIC**: Soothing music is music that is relaxing and calming to listen to.

248. **SPIRITUAL AWAKENING**: Spiritual awakening is a profound shift in consciousness or awareness often associated with personal growth and enlightenment.

249. **STIMULATES CREATIVITY**: Stimulates creativity means to inspire or enhance the ability to generate new ideas or artistic expressions.

250. **STRESS MANAGEMENT**: Stress management involves strategies and techniques to cope with and reduce stress.

251. **STRESS RESPONSE**: The stress response is the body's physiological reaction to stressors, often involving increased heart rate, release of stress hormones, and heightened alertness.

252. **SUBTLE ENERGY**: Subtle energy refers to the energy that is not easily measurable but is believed to exist in various spiritual and alternative healing traditions.

253. **SUNSTONE**: Sunstone is a type of gemstone known for its bright and reflective appearance, often used in jewelry.

254. **SYMBIOTIC RELATIONSHIPS**: Symbiotic relationships are mutually beneficial partnerships between different organisms.

255. **SYNCHRONICITIES**: Synchronicities are meaningful coincidences that seem to be connected by more than just chance.

256. **SYNERGISTIC EFFECTS**: Synergistic effects are interactions between different elements that result in a combined effect greater than the sum of their individual effects.

257. **SYNTHESIZED**: Synthesized means created by combining different elements or components.

258. **TENSION RELEASE**: Tension release involves methods and practices that help relax and relieve physical or emotional tension.

259. **THERAPEUTIC**: Therapeutic means having healing or medicinal properties or benefits.

260. **THERAPEUTIC MODALITIES**: Therapeutic modalities are various methods and approaches used for healing and well-being.

261. **TISSUE REGENERATION**: Tissue regeneration is the process of repairing and replacing damaged or lost tissues in the body.

262. **TRANSCENDENTAL MEDITATION**: Transcendental Meditation is a specific form of meditation that aims to reach a unique state of restful awareness.

263. **TRANSCENDENTAL STATES**: Transcendental states are altered states of consciousness that go beyond ordinary awareness.

264. **TRANSCENDS**: Transcends means to go beyond or surpass something.

265. **TRANSFORMATIONAL EXPERIENCES**: Transformational experiences are events or moments that lead to significant personal change or growth.

266. **TRANSFORMATIVE**: Transformative means causing a profound or significant change.

267. **TURMERIC**: Turmeric is a bright yellow spice with potential health benefits and is commonly used in cooking.

268. **UNPRECEDENTED**: Unprecedented means never before seen or experienced.

269. **UPREGULATE**: Upregulate means to increase or enhance the activity or expression of something, often used in biological contexts.

270. **UPRIGHT POSTURE**: Upright posture refers to standing or sitting with the body in a straight and balanced position.

271. **VAGUS NERVE**: The vagus nerve is a cranial nerve that plays a crucial role in regulating various bodily functions, including digestion and heart rate.

272. **VALERIAN ROOT**: Valerian root is an herbal supplement known for its potential calming and sleep-inducing effects.

273. **VITAL ENERGY**: Vital energy, often referred to as "qi" or "prana," is believed to be the life force that flows through living beings.

274. **VITAL FORCE**: Vital force is the energy or spirit that animates living organisms.

275. **VITAMINS**: Vitamins are essential nutrients needed by the body for various functions, often obtained through diet or supplements.

276. **WELL-BEING**: Well-being is a state of overall health, happiness, and prosperity.

277. **WHITE QUARTZ**: White quartz is a type of crystal known for its clarity and purity, often used in jewelry and metaphysical practices.

278. **WISDOM TRADITIONS**: Wisdom traditions are ancient or cultural practices and teachings that impart knowledge about life and spirituality.

279. **YLANG-YLANG**: Ylang-ylang is a fragrant flower known for its aromatic oil, often used in perfumes and aromatherapy.

280. **YOGA**: Yoga is a physical, mental, and spiritual practice that aims to promote physical strength, flexibility, relaxation, and inner peace.

I hope you find these definitions helpful! If you have any more words or questions, feel free to ask.

REFERENCES

1. **https://www.ncbi.nlm.nih.gov/pmc/articles/PMC4378297/:** This is a PubMed article that discusses the effects of grounding on inflammation, immune response, wound healing, and prevention and treatment of chronic inflammatory and autoimmune diseases.

2. **https://earthinginstitute.net/what-is-earthing/:** This website provides a brief overview of Earthing (grounding) and its benefits. It explains how Earthing works and how it can help reduce inflammation, pain, and stress.

3. **https://dovemedicalpress.altmetric.com/details/3889821/facebook:** This Altmetric article refers to the same PubMed article mentioned in the first source. The article highlights the interesting research on "grounding" and the effect it can have on inflammation, immune response, wound healing, and prevention and treatment of chronic inflammatory and autoimmune diseases.

4. **https://www.ncbi.nlm.nih.gov/pmc/articles/pmc4378297/:** This is the same PubMed article mentioned in the first and third sources. It discusses the effects of grounding on inflammation, immune response, wound healing, and prevention and treatment of chronic inflammatory and autoimmune diseases.

5. **https://www.researchgate.net/publication/274644091_The_effects_of_grounding_earthing_on_inflammation_the_immune_response_wound_healing_and_prevention_and_treatment_of_chronic_inflammatory_and_autoimmu**

ne_diseases: This is a ResearchGate article that discusses the effects of grounding on inflammation, immune response, wound healing, and prevention and treatment of chronic inflammatory and autoimmune diseases.

6. https://www.nfpa.org/News-and-Research/Publications-and-media/Blogs-Landing-Page/NFPA-Today/Blog-Posts/2021/09/27/Grounding-Understanding-the-Essentials-for-Building-the-Foundation-of-a-Structures-Electrical-System: This website provides an overview of grounding in the context of building and structure electrical systems. It explains the importance of grounding and how it stabilizes voltage and helps clear ground faults.

7. https://dovemedicalpress.altmetric.com/details/3889821/facebook: This Altmetric article refers to the same PubMed article mentioned in the first source. The article highlights the interesting research on "grounding" and the effect it can have on inflammation, immune response, wound healing, and prevention and treatment of chronic inflammatory and autoimmune diseases.

8. https://www.ncbi.nlm.nih.gov/pmc/articles/pmc4378297/: This is the same PubMed article mentioned in the first and third sources. It discusses the effects of grounding on inflammation, immune response, wound healing, and prevention and treatment of chronic inflammatory and autoimmune diseases.

9. https://www.researchgate.net/publication/274644091_The_effects_of_grounding_earthing_on_inflammation_the_immune_response_wound_healing_and_prevention_and_treatment_of_chronic_inflammatory_and_autoimmune_diseases: This is a ResearchGate article that discusses

the effects of grounding on inflammation, immune response, wound healing, and prevention and treatment of chronic inflammatory and autoimmune diseases.

10. **https://www.nfpa.org/News-and-Research/Publications-and-media/Blogs-Landing-Page/NFPA-Today/Blog-Posts/2021/09/27/Grounding-Understanding-the-Essentials-for-Building-the-Foundation-of-a-Structures-Electrical-System:** This website provides an overview of grounding in the context of building and structure electrical systems. It explains the importance of grounding and how it stabilizes voltage and helps clear ground faults.

11. **https://store.samhsa.gov/sites/default/files/d7/priv/pep19-01-01-005.pdf:** This is a PDF document that provides guidance on communicating in a crisis. It highlights the importance of sound and thoughtful risk communication in preventing ineffective, fear-driven, and potentially damaging public responses to serious situations.

12. **https://www.helpscout.com/customer-service-examples/:** This website provides 12 customer service response templates and examples to craft your own replies to tricky support requests. One of the templates provided is a response for when you don't have access to the information the customer is requesting. The template suggests redirecting the customer to the appropriate support team and providing them with helpful information to include in their request.

13. **https://store.samhsa.gov/sites/default/files/d7/priv/pep19-01-01-005.pdf:** This is a PDF document that provides guidance on communicating in a crisis. It highlights the importance of sound and thoughtful risk communication

in preventing ineffective, fear-driven, and potentially damaging public responses to serious situations.

14. **https://www.sciencedirect.com/science/article/pii/s2319417022001524:** This is a ScienceDirect article that discusses the effects of grounding on the human body. The article highlights that grounding can reduce inflammation, improve sleep, and reduce stress and anxiety.

15. **https://www.helpscout.com/customer-service-examples/:** This website provides 12 customer service response templates and examples to craft your own replies to tricky support requests. One of the templates provided is a response for when you don't have access to the information the customer is requesting. The template suggests redirecting the customer to the appropriate support team and providing them with helpful information to include in their request.

ABOUT THE AUTHOR

Harkeem Shaw is a man of many talents, including being a veteran, aeronautical engineer, information technician, and author. He is also a passionate advocate for the importance of grounding to one's well-being. Shaw's diverse background has given him a unique perspective on the intersection of science and spirituality, particularly the ways in which the human body interacts with the natural world. His book, Earthing: The Hidden Power of Grounding Yourself, explores the scientific evidence behind the benefits of grounding. Grounding is the practice of connecting the human body to the earth's electrical field, which Shaw argues can have a number of health benefits, including reducing inflammation, improving sleep quality, boosting energy levels, and relieving chronic pain. He also discusses the spiritual and emotional benefits of grounding, such as its ability to reduce stress and anxiety and promote a sense of well-being. Shaw's work has helped to raise awareness of the importance of grounding to human health and well-being, and he is the founder of The Grounding Factory, LLC, an organization that promotes the practice of grounding and provides educational resources and support to individuals and organizations interested in learning more about grounding and its benefits. Shaw's work is a testament to the power of science and spirituality to work together to improve our well-being, and he is a role model for all of us who are passionate about living a healthy and balanced life.

Made in the USA
Monee, IL
09 September 2024